RADIOLOGY FOR UNDERGRADUATE
FINALS AND FOUNDATION

Key topics and questions

RADIOLOGY FOR UNDERGRADUATE FINALS AND FOUNDATION YEARS

Key topics and question types

TRISTAN BARRETT

Radiology Registrar
Addenbrooke's Hospital, Cambridge

NADEEM SHAIDA

Radiology Registrar
Addenbrooke's Hospital, Cambridge

and

ASHLEY SHAW

Consultant Radiologist
Addenbrooke's Hospital, Cambridge

Foreword by

ADRIAN K DIXON

Professor of Radiology
University of Cambridge

Radcliffe Publishing
Oxford • New York

Radcliffe Publishing Ltd
18 Marcham Road
Abingdon
Oxon OX14 1AA
United Kingdom

www.radcliffepublishing.com
Electronic catalogue and worldwide online ordering facility.

British Library Cataloguing in Publication Data

A catalogue record for this book is available from the British Library.

ISBN-13: 978 184619 446 7

The paper used for the text pages of this book
is FSC certified. FSC (The Forest Stewardship
Council) is an international network to promote
responsible management of the world's forests.

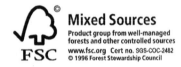

Mixed Sources
Product group from well-managed
forests and other controlled sources
www.fsc.org Cert no. SGS-COC-2482
© 1996 Forest Stewardship Council

Typeset by Phoenix Photosetting, Chatham, Kent
Printed and bound by TJI Digital, Padstow, Cornwall

Contents

Foreword

It is a great honour to be asked to provide a foreword for this excellent and unusual text which is predominantly aimed at senior medical students and those doctors who are taking examinations in their early years of postgraduate medicine. It is one of the first books specifically designed for new ways of teaching with extended matching item (EMI), objective structured clinical examination (OSCE) questions as well as more conventional MCQs, both in the form of single best answer questions and more conventional True or False questions. There are also useful pointers as to likely viva questions in all examinations and interviews.

There is an eminently practical range of topics covered in this book and this reflects the commonsense approach by the authors. The images are good and the explanatory text educationally valuable and very much to the point.

It is not the sort of book that one would use as an initial textbook in the subject but it should prove invaluable about a year and a half before final examinations. As a quick revision before MRCP or MRCS and other postgraduate examinations, it would also be very useful. Furthermore it would be very much in a candidate's interest to be familiar with the contents before attending an interview process for a radiology specialist registrar post. Although designed for the UK market it has just as many applications in European countries and further afield. I very much hope that the authors see success with this book. They have put a lot of effort into it on behalf of medical students and doctors in training.

Adrian K Dixon
Professor of Radiology, University of Cambridge
Honorary Consultant Radiologist, Addenbrooke's Hospital, Cambridge
July 2010

Preface

Radiology as a medical specialty has expanded in recent times due to advances in technology and in the quality of images that can be produced. This has resulted in a countrywide increase in posts, investment in equipment and PACS systems to meet demand, and increasing representation of the specialty in the medical school curriculum. The majority of in-patients will undergo some form of imaging during their admission, ranging from plain film through to CT and MRI. Thus, for the medical student soon to become a post-graduate practicing doctor, regardless of the specialty entered into, basic knowledge of radiology is essential: when to investigate a patient, which modality is best to answer a specific clinical question, how to interpret a chest and abdominal plain film.

Thus radiology now forms a firm part of all clinical year assessments and, in particular, the final examinations; this book addresses the different ways in which the subject can be assessed. Additionally, the basics of radiology are introduced including the physics behind the images, a 'rough-guide' to the modalities used, and the future directions in the field.

Tristan Barrett
Nadeem Shaida
Ashley Shaw
July 2010

About the authors

Tristan Barrett is currently a radiology registrar at Addenbrooke's Hospital, Cambridge. He qualified in 2002, and gained MRCP membership in 2005. Two years research experience at National Institutes for Health, Bethesda, USA led to numerous publications in radiology journals. He has also been the primary author for several invited chapters published in radiology text books.

Nadeem Shaida graduated from St Bartholomew's and The Royal London School of Medicine in 2000. After gaining the MRCS examination in 2004, he commenced radiology training in 2007 at Addenbrooke's Hospital in Cambridge. He has previously published in a variety of areas within medicine including a previous book aimed at radiology trainees. His current interests include interventional and oncological radiology.

Ashley Shaw trained in radiology at King's College Hospital, London. He is currently a consultant radiologist at Addenbrooke's Hospital, Cambridge, having been appointed in 2004. Research interests include transplantation, oncology, and cross-sectional imaging.

List of abbreviations

A&E	Accident and emergency
AAA	Abdominal aortic aneurysm
ABPA	Allergic bronchopulmonary aspergillosis
ACA	Anterior cerebral artery
ACE	Angiotensin converting enzyme
ACTH	Adrenocorticotropic hormone
ALARP	As low as reasonably practicable
ALP	Alkaline phosphatase
ALT	Alanine transaminase
AP	Antero-posterior
ARDS	Adult respiratory distress syndrome
AS	Ankylosing spondylitis
AVM	Arteriovenous malformation
AVN	Avascular necrosis
AXR	Abdominal X-ray
BGS	British Gastroenterology Society
BP	Blood pressure
BRCA	Breast cancer gene
BS	Bone scintigram
CBD	Common bile duct
CC	Cranio-caudal
CCF	Congestive cardiac failure
CF	Cystic fibrosis
CHD	Congenital heart disease
CNS	Central nervous system
CMCJ	Carpo-metacarpal joint
CMV	Cytomegalovirus
COPD	Chronic obstructive pulmonary disease
CSF	Cerebro-spinal fluid
CT	Computed tomography
CTA	Computed tomography angiography
CTKUB	Computed tomography kidneys ureter bladder
CTPA	Computed tomography pulmonary angiography
CVS	Chorionic villus sampling

CXR	Chest X-ray
D&C	Dilatation and curettage
DCE-MRI	Dynamic contrast-enhanced magnetic resonance imaging
DCIS	Ductal carcinoma in situ
DCM	Dilated cardiomyopathy
DDH	Developmental dysplasia of the hip
DEXA	Dual energy X-ray absorptiometry
DGH	District general hospital
DHS	Dynamic hip screw
DIC	Disseminated intravascular coagulation
DIPJ	Distal interphalangeal joint
DMSA	Dimercaptosuccinic acid
DNA	Deoxyribonucleic acid
DSA	Digital subtraction angiography
DTPA	Diethylene triamine pentaacetic acid
DVT	Deep vein thrombosis
DWI	Diffusion weighted imaging
EAA	Extrinsic allergic alveolitis
ECMO	Extracorporal membrane oxygenation
EDH	Extra-dural haematoma
EDTA	Ethylenediaminetetraacetic acid
ERCP	Endoscopic retrograde cholangiopancreatogram
ESR	Erythrocyte sedimentation rate
EUS	Endoscopic ultrasound
FAST	Focused assessment with sonography for trauma
FBC	Full blood count
FDG	Fluoro-deoxy-glucose
FNA	Fine needle aspiration
GCS	Glasgow coma scale
GFR	Glomerular filtration rate
GI	Gastrointestinal
GP	General practitioner
GOJ	Gastro-oesophageal junction
Hb	Haemoglobin
HHT	Hereditary haemorrhagic telangiectasia
HMD	Hyaline membrane disease
HOA	Hypertrophic osteoarthropathy
HPOA	Hypertrophic pulmonary osteoarthropathy
HPT	Hyperparathyroidism
HRCT	High resolution computed tomography
HSG	Hysterosalpingogram
HU	Hounsfield units
IBD	Inflammatory bowel disease
ICP	Intracranial pressure
IDA	Iron deficiency anaemia
IgE	Immunoglobulin E
IPJ	Interphalangeal joint

IR(ME)R	Ionising radiation (medical exposure) regulations
IUGR	Intrauterine growth retardation
i.v.	Intravenous
IVC	Inferior vena cava
IVU	Intravenous urogram
KUB	Kidneys ureter bladder X-ray
LAM	Lymphangioleiomyomatosis
LBO	Large bowel obstruction
LCH	Langerhans cell histiocytosis
LDH	Lactate dehydrogenase
LES	Lower (o)esophageal sphincter
LFT	Liver function tests
LIP	Lymphocytic interstitial pneumonia
LLL	Left lower lobe
LP	Lumbar puncture
LUL	Left upper lobe
LVF	Left ventricular failure
MAG-3	Mercapto acetyl tri-glycine
MCA	Middle cerebral artery
MCPJ	Metacarpo-phalangeal joint
MCUG	Micturating cystourogram
MCV	Mean corpuscular volume
MDP	Methyl diphosphonate
MDT	Multi-disciplinary team
MEN	Multiple endocrine neoplasia
MHz	Megahertz
MI	Myocardial infarction
MIBG	Meta-iodobenzylguanidine
MLO	Medial-lateral oblique view
MRA	Magnetic resonance angiography
MRCP	Magnetic resonance cholangiopancreatogram
MRI	Magnetic resonance imaging
MRSA	Methicillin-resistant staphylococcus aureus
mSv	Millisieverts
MTPJ	Metatarso-phalangeal joint
NAI	Non accidental injury
NEC	Necrotising enterocolitis
NF	Neurofibromatosis
NICE	National Institute for Clinical Excellence
NJ	Naso-jejunal
NPH	Normal pressure hydrocephalus
NSAID	Non-steroidal anti-inflammatory drug
NSIP	Non-specific interstitial pneumonia
NSF	Nephrogenic systemic fibrosis
OA	Osteoarthritis
OCP	Oral contraceptive pill
OGD	Oesophago-gastroduodenoscopy

OSCE	Objective structured clinical examination
PA	Posterior-anterior view
PACS	Picture archiving and communications system
PAN	Polyarteritis nodosa
PAVM	Pulmonary arteriovenous malformation
PCD	Primary ciliary dyskinesia
PCP	Pneumocystis carinii pneumonia
PDA	Patent ductus arteriosus
PE	Pulmonary embolus
PEG	Percutaneous endoscopic gastrostomy
PET	Positron emission tomography
PIPJ	Proximal interphalangeal joint
PR	Per rectum
PSA	Prostate specific antigen
PSC	Primary sclerosing cholangitis
PTC	Percutaneous transhepatic cholangiography
PTH	Parathyroid hormone
PV	Per vagina
RCR	Royal College of Radiologists
RDS	Respiratory distress syndrome
RhA	Rheumatoid arthritis
RIF	Right iliac fossa
RIG	Radiologically inserted gastrostomy
RLL	Right lower lobe
RLZ	Right lower zone
RML	Right middle lobe
RSV	Respiratory syncytial virus
RTA	Road traffic accident
RUL	Right upper lobe
RUQ	Right upper quadrant
SAH	Subarachnoid haemorrhage
SBO	Small bowel obstruction
SCC	Squamous cell carcinoma
SCD	Sickle cell disease
SDH	Subdural haematoma
SI	Sacro-iliac
SLE	Systemic lupus erythematosus
SUFE	Slipped upper femoral epiphysis
SVC	Superior vena cava
TB	Tuberculosis
TCC	Transitional cell carcinoma
TIA	Transient ischaemic attack
TS	Tuberous sclerosis
TTN	Transient tachypnoea of the newborn
TV	Trans vaginal
U&E	Urea and electrolytes
UC	Ulcerative colitis

UIP	Usual interstitial pneumonia
US	Ultrasound
UTI	Urinary tract infection
VHL	von Hippel-Lindau
V/Q	Ventilation/perfusion scan
WCC	White cell count

Chapter 1
Introduction

RADIOLOGY: A BRIEF HISTORY

The 'birth' of radiology can be considered as being in 1895 with the discovery of X-rays, by German physicist Wilhelm Conrad Röntgen. The 'X-rays' he produced are still referred to by some as 'Röntgen rays', or the English language version 'Roentgen rays', in his honour. Soon after their discovery, X-rays were being used for various applications including fitting shoes, and diagnostic medical imaging. Initially, a variety of hospital personnel conducted radiography including physicists, photographers, doctors, nurses, and engineers. The medical specialty of radiology grew up over many years around the new technology. The origins of the British Institute of Radiology (BIR) can be traced back to a first meeting held on 2 April 1897 to form 'The X-ray Society'. The first general meeting of the new society renamed 'The Röntgen Society' in honour of Wilhelm Röntgen, was held on 3 June 1897. Eventually, as the technique evolved, the Society of Radiographers was formed in 1920, and from the 1930s doctors were appointed with a specific interest in the use of X-rays for diagnosis or therapy, thus the specialty of radiology was formed.

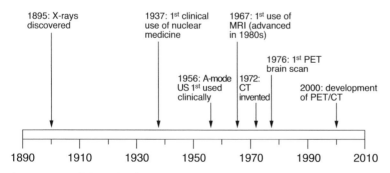

Figure 1.1 Radiology timeline.

AN EVOLVING SPECIALTY

The practice of medicine and surgery has changed immeasurably in recent years with an increasing reliance on diagnostic tests, whether they are biochemical, haematological, or radiological. Patients are better informed and have greater expectations than ever before. Consequently, it is crucial that clinicians have a basic understanding of radiology in order that they can optimise investigations, understand the risks and benefits of different studies, interpret basic investigations and be able to communicate effectively with their patients about these in the clinic or the ward situation.

In response to these developments, radiology has been increasingly incorporated into the medical school curriculum through lectures and film-based teaching. Radiology lends itself very well to examinations and these can take many forms, from multiple choice questions through to the objective structured clinical examination (OSCE) and the viva voce.

The aim of the first sections of this book is to provide medical students with a basic knowledge of the radiology department. What do the tests involve? What issues do I need to consider? What is the radiation dose? How should I present the radiological image? The later chapters aim to educate the reader through the various types of questions that may be encountered: OSCE questions, multiple choice questions, single best answer questions, short answer questions, extended matching items, and viva topics. Each question has a full answer, and the book covers a broad range of radiological topics that one might encounter at this stage of medical education.

Chapter 2
The radiology imaging modalities

X-RAYS/FLUOROSCOPY

X-rays are high energy electromagnetic waves. In diagnostic radiology, they are emitted from a point source, directed through the relevant part of the body and onto a radiographic plate (previously a film). As they pass through the body, X-rays are absorbed to different degrees by different tissues, which is dependent upon their density and thickness, i.e. bone absorbs more than soft tissue, which in turn absorbs more than air. This gives the appearance of white for bone, black for air and grey for the soft tissues when viewed. Fluoroscopy uses continuous low dose X-rays to give a moving image and can be used to give functional information, for example in the evaluation of the GI tract.

Main uses:

- Chest X-ray.
- Abdominal X-ray.
- Extremity films: fractures, arthritis.
- Barium fluoroscopy studies.
- Interventional fluoroscopy (*see* below).
- Mammography.

Advantages	Disadvantages
Relatively low radiation dose	Poor soft tissue differentiation
Quick	Generally poor sensitivity and specificity
Cheap	
Available	

COMPUTED TOMOGRAPHY

Computed tomography (CT) comprises a gantry housing an X-ray tube, a bank of detectors, and a table on which the patient lies. The patient moves through the gantry as the X-ray tube and detectors rotate around them at high speed. This creates a three-dimensional volume of data within a matter of seconds that can be reconstructed to provide images in any plane. CT uses high doses of ionising radiation to achieve these images, typically up to 10 milli-Sieverts (mSv), the equivalent of around three years of background radiation. Therefore, it is crucial to weigh the risks and benefits of the procedure in each case. CT is widely used to image the brain, thorax, abdomen and pelvis, enabling rapid imaging of even the sickest patient.

Main uses:

- Head injury.
- Abdominal / chest trauma.
- Detection and staging of malignancy.
- Investigation of the acute abdomen.

Advantages	Disadvantages
Excellent spatial resolution	Ionising radiation
Available	Nephrotoxicity of iodinated contrast media
Linear relationship of contrast dose allows characterisation of lesion content	High volume of images for the radiologist to interpret
High sensitivity and specificity	Cost
Multi-planar reconstruction	
Quick	

ULTRASOUND

Ultrasound (US) uses sound waves of 2–15 MHz (above the range of human hearing) to produce images. The ultrasound probe acts as both emitter and receiver of the ultrasound waves in order to create an image. Ultrasound does not utilise any ionising radiation and is considered safe in pregnancy and for use in children, although there is a theoretical risk from the heating of tissues. Ultrasound has many applications and may be used to image the brain (neonates), soft tissues, peripheral vascular system, abdomen and pelvis, as well as the developing foetus. The major limitations of ultrasound are its inability to pass through air (lung, colon) or bone. In obese patients, abdominal or pelvic US may be limited by the depth of penetration of the sound waves.

Main uses:

- Renal tract imaging.
- Biliary imaging / cholecystitis.
- Liver imaging / lesion characterisation.
- Deep vein thrombosis.
- Doppler imaging: carotid stenoses; AAA; post liver / renal transplant vascularity.
- Gynaecological imaging.
- Musculoskeletal imaging.
- Others: breast, thyroid, testes.

Advantages	Disadvantages
Available	Operator dependent
Portable	Limited depth penetration
Non-invasive	Limited anatomical access: US waves cannot penetrate through bone or air
No ionising radiation	Patient factors: e.g. liver high under the rib cage; limited in obesity
Real-time imaging (e.g. biopsies)	

MAGNETIC RESONANCE IMAGING

Magnetic resonance imaging (MRI) involves placing a patient on a table in a relatively confined space (often described by patients as a tunnel) within a strong magnetic field. This causes some alignment of the hydrogen atoms within the body along the magnetic field. A series of radiofrequency waves are then used to displace these atoms and, as they return to their original positions, they emit a small radiofrequency signal. An image is constructed from these signals – essentially a map of hydrogen atoms. However, the signal varies according to the local milieu and hence MRI can differentiate soft tissues. MRI is used extensively for the brain and central nervous system, musculoskeletal evaluation, and abdominal and pelvic imaging. The relatively narrow bore and safety considerations within the magnet make imaging the acutely unwell patient particularly difficult. Imaging patients with cardiac devices is contraindicated, whilst ferromagnetic objects in the body (e.g. shrapnel) may move or become heated during an examination. Of crucial importance, if called to attend an emergency within an MRI department, one should not enter the magnetic field without express permission of the radiographers.

Main uses:

- Musculoskeletal imaging.
- Neuro imaging: stroke, lesion characterisation.
- Liver imaging: lesion characterisation.
- MRCP.
- Gynaecological imaging.
- Spinal cord / intervertebral disc imaging.

Advantages	Disadvantages
No ionising radiation	Movement artefact (e.g. respiratory motion in chest)
Excellent soft tissue differentiation	Susceptibility artefact (e.g. metallic implants)
Gadolinium agents have a better toxicity profile than CT contrast agents	Patient unsuitability: claustrophobia / pacemakers
Functional imaging: diffusion-weighting, spectroscopy	Less spatial resolution than CT
	Availability
	High volume of images for the radiologist to interpret
	Cost
	Length of examination

NUCLEAR MEDICINE

Nuclear medicine differs from other forms of imaging in many ways. The radiation source is inside the patient, having been injected or ingested. The radiation source is a combination of a radioactive nuclide and a molecule which has a metabolic function, i.e. the aim is to incorporate the radionuclide into a physiological process and monitor it by measuring / imaging the radioactivity. The process uses gamma-rays, electromagnetic waves of higher energy than X-rays, which are then detected by either a ring or panel of detectors. As a consequence of not having a point source, the spatial resolution is less than in other forms of radiology, but the functional information provided may be more revealing.

Recently, hybrid imaging has been introduced. This combines functional imaging with a CT machine and enables the fusion and correlation of functional and anatomical data. Perhaps the best known example of this is positron emission tomography (PET-CT). This typically uses radioactive fluoride in a molecule that mimics glucose. As such, it provides a metabolic map of the body and is increasingly being used in the field of oncology in particular.

Main uses:

- V/Q scans for PE.
- Bone scans for bone lesions.
- Functional renal imaging.
- PET-CT for oncology staging.
- Thyroid imaging / treatment.
- Dynamic cardiac imaging.
- WCC for occult infection.

Advantages	Disadvantages
High sensitivity	Ionising radiation
Provides functional information	Low specificity
Quantification possible	Poor spatial resolution for anatomical correlation
Treatment of thyroid disease	Availability (need specialist radiochemistry, cyclotrons, etc., to produce tracers)
	Risk of public and staff radiation exposure
	Scanners are mildly claustrophobic
	Time taken: e.g. bone scan requires patient to return at 4 hours

INTERVENTIONAL RADIOLOGY

Interventional radiology is a broad term covering a range of diagnostic and therapeutic procedures which can be divided into vascular and non-vascular. Vascular procedures are primarily therapeutic (with diagnosis being performed increasingly by CT or MRI) and include line placement, angioplasty and stent insertion. Perhaps the greatest advance in this field over the past decade has been the treatment of aortic aneurysms by endovascular means, avoiding the need for open surgery. Non-vascular intervention includes procedures of the liver and biliary tract, gastrointestinal or urinary tract. These procedures use fluoroscopy to guide the radiologist.

INTERPRETING RADIOLOGICAL IMAGES

Whether as a student in an examination situation or a practising clinician, there are a number of basic rules to follow when looking at radiological images.

- Check the patient's name is correct.
- Check the date of the study.

- Ensure that you have all the relevant images available.
- Confirm the image is orientated correctly.

These rules may seem self-explanatory, but with the increasing use of Patient Archiving and Communications Systems (PACS), it is very easy to look at the wrong patient or image. Images may be in different files and you may inadvertently invert the image – always check the markers.

The extremity films – a special case

When looking at images of the extremities (bones and joints), there are several points to remember:

- At least two views should be obtained for most indications.
- Fractures or dislocations may only be visible on one view.
- Fracture terminology (*see* below) describes the distal fragment in relation to the proximal fragment.
- In arthritis, it is important to pay attention to the distribution of disease.

Fracture terminology can be confusing, but there are basic rules that apply. Generally long bones are divided into 'thirds' (proximal, middle, or distal) to describe the fracture location, alternatively, anatomical landmarks can be used.

- Comminuted: three or more fragments are present.
- Compact (open): the skin surface is breached; a clinical finding.
- Fracture line: transverse, oblique, or spiral.
- Longitudinal length: reduced (overlapping bones; 'impacted'), or increased (distraction).
- Displacement: lateral / medial / anterior / posterior / volar / dorsal.
- Joints: subluxation means there remains some apposition of the joints; dislocation means there is none.

THE CHEST X-RAY

The chest film is perhaps one of the most common radiological investigations performed, but its interpretation is difficult to master. The key is to simplify – practice a routine for evaluating the image and describe the signs fully before delivering a (differential) diagnosis. The more films you see (both normal and abnormal), the more confident you will become in identifying abnormalities and describing the film. A simple routine would be:

- Technique (erect or supine, PA or PA).
- Lines, tubes and devices.
- Heart size (PA film only).
- Mediastinal contours.
- Lungs (comparing left with right).
- Pleura (costophrenic recesses).
- Bones.
- Soft tissues.
- Look below the diaphragm.

THE ABDOMINAL X-RAY

If looking at abdominal films, there are a few things to mention:

- Is the bowel calibre normal?
- Is the mucosal pattern normal?
- Is there free air?
- Presence of any calcification.

CT IMAGES

When looking at CT studies, these will usually be presented in the axial (transverse plane). By convention, these are viewed as if looking up from the patient's feet. When assessing a CT image or study, consider the following:

- What part of the body has been imaged?
- What window settings have been used (lung, soft tissue, brain, bone)?
- Has the patient been given contrast medium, orally or i.v.?
- Look at each organ in turn and describe abnormalities before drawing conclusions.
- In the brain and lungs, compare left with right.

MR IMAGING

MRI studies can be difficult to approach without much experience. However, there are a few pointers which may be helpful:

- Describe the site of imaging.
- Describe the plane of imaging (axial, sagittal, coronal).
- T1-weighted imaging (fluid is dark); this sequence is best for anatomical detail.
- T2-weighted imaging (fluid is bright); this sequence is best for identifying pathology.
- Fat or water may have been suppressed to increase the contrast in the image.
- Imaging following i.v. gadolinium is performed with T1-weighted sequences.

Chapter 3

Key topics in radiology: contrast media, radiation protection and the future of radiology

CONTRAST MEDIA

Contrast media are used within all areas of radiology to provide additional information. Their physical properties may be used to increase the contrast between adjacent structures and to provide functional information about an organ or lesion.

Barium-based contrast medium has been used for many years in the investigation of the gastrointestinal tract. It has a high density and thus absorbs more X-rays than adjacent soft tissues. Barium studies have been increasingly replaced by endoscopy, CT and MRI in recent years. Barium stimulates a chemical peritonitis if it spills into the peritoneal cavity which has a 50% mortality, hence, it is contraindicated in patients with suspected bowel perforation or anastomotic leaks. Barium can also cause a chemical pneumonitis if aspirated, but this usually only requires chest physiotherapy.

Iodine-based contrast medium has a variety of forms that may be administered by oral, rectal, intravascular and every other conceivable route, depending on the agent. Iodine has a high density and thus absorbs more X-rays than soft tissues. When given in the GI tract, the lumen will be demonstrated, when administered via an intravascular route, the contrast medium will enhance the vessels and subsequently the various tissues within the body. It improves differentiation of adjacent soft tissue structures with different enhancement characteristics. More recently, functional CT imaging enables the radiologist to determine more accurately the rate of blood flow, blood volume, and transit time across an organ. There are two principal concerns with iodinated contrast medium: allergic reactions and contrast induced nephropathy. When a patient has an injection of iodine-based contrast medium, they experience a hot flush, may feel nauseous and feel a need to urinate.

A small proportion of patients will show allergic symptoms ranging from an urticarial rash through to a life-threatening anaphylactoid reaction. It is important to include this information when requesting a CT study. Patients may experience a transient deterioration in renal function following the administration of intravenous contrast medium. This is usually insignificant and renal function returns to normal. However, patients with impaired renal function may suffer a significant deterioration that might require renal support and this complication can be devastating for the patient. Therefore, in patients with known renal failure, very careful consideration should be given before administering intravenous contrast medium, balancing the risks and benefits to the patient. Good hydration and careful fluid balance is crucial in this situation. This is not an issue for end-stage renal failure patients on haemodialysis, as the dialysis will remove the contrast agent.

In MRI, gadolinium is utilised as an intravenous contrast agent. Gadolinium alters the magnetic properties of tissues and, following injection, may increase the contrast between adjacent tissues. Additionally, an organ may be imaged repeatedly to provide dynamic images which can give functional information about an organ or lesion. Over the past decade, there has been increasing recognition that gadolinium may cause nephrogenic systemic fibrosis (NSF) when given to patients with renal failure. NSF is a rare but potentially fatal multi-system disorder that may affect the skin or solid organs. As such gadolinium is contraindicated in patients with renal failure.

Ultrasound contrast medium is used in some centres, but not all. It comprises 'microbubbles' with a diameter of 1 μm to 10 μm, formed from a thin layer of albumin, lipid, or polymer and containing a gas such as a perfluorocarbon or nitrogen. These agents are injected intravenously and remain in the intravascular space. The microbubbles resonate at the frequencies used in diagnostic ultrasound and this makes them effective reflectors. They may be used to demonstrate the vascularity of focal lesions within solid organs or to evaluate the vessels themselves. Hypersensitivity to these agents is possible, but there are no other complications associated.

IONISING RADIATION CONSIDERATIONS

Both X-rays and gamma rays are high energy electromagnetic waves which, on interacting with matter, deposit a variable amount of energy. This may result in the ionisation of atoms or molecules which, in a living organism, may ultimately result in damage to the structure and function of a cell or its DNA. The consequences of ionising radiation upon a living organism may be divided into two categories. Those effects that have a threshold dose, which are predictable and directly related to dose, for example skin burns, alopecia or radiation sickness, are termed deterministic. Effects that may or may not happen, for example the development of cancer, are termed stochastic. Whilst the probability of a stochastic effect increases with dose, there is no threshold below which they do not occur, i.e. there is no safe dose of radiation. In diagnostic radiology the latter is of greater concern as the doses used rarely approach the threshold necessary for deterministic effects.

Every day, we are exposed to background radiation from a number of different sources, arising predominantly from radon gas, the earth, from space, medical sources and even in our food. A tiny amount (< 0.5%) comes from weapons discharge and radioactive waste disposal. The level of background radiation that we experience depends on where we live. In the UK, the average level is 2.64 mSv (including medical exposures), but this increases to 7.44 mSv in Cornwall, due to high levels of radon gas. Similarly, one is exposed to increased radiation when flying; a round-trip from London to New York would have an approximate additional exposure of 0.1 mSv, equivalent to five chest radiographs.

Increasingly, patients are likely to express concern regarding exposure to medical radiation. When discussing these issues with patients, it is often best to compare the radiation doses against the natural background exposure. A table of common investigations with approximate doses is given below. In addition, patients often ask about the risk of developing cancer. Epidemiological studies are largely based on high dose exposures, particularly the atomic bombs deployed at the end of the Second World War. The best estimates suggest the risk of a single CT study varies from 1 in 1000 to 1 in 10 000, depending upon the patient's age,[1] but it is impossible to observe the effects at this level directly due to the high background prevalence of cancer.

Procedure	Dose (mSv)	Approx equivalent UK background radiation
Extremity X-ray	0.001	<1 day
Chest X-ray	0.02	3 days
Mammography	0.7	3 months
Abdominal X-ray	1	5 months
CT head	2	11 months
CT abdomen or pelvis	4–6	2–3 years
CT chest, abdomen and pelvis	10	4.5 years
Bone scintigraphy	4	2 years
PET-CT	10–12	4.5–6 years

FUTURE DIRECTIONS IN RADIOLOGY

Traditionally, imaging modalities have been used to provide anatomical imaging; any imaging technique which affords information on function within the region scanned is broadly classified as 'functional imaging'. The main imaging modalities of US, MRI and CT are reaching the upper limit of their obtainable resolution: any further improvement in CT resolution will involve an unacceptable increase in radiation dose, whilst, aside from coil development and higher strength magnets (which also raises safety concerns), major MRI improvements can only be achieved by increasing scan times (hence reduced patient 'through put' and worse patient compliance). As a result future advances in imaging are likely to be based on the development of functional techniques or functional imaging agents, or the use of multi-modality scanning.

All nuclear medicine studies involve an element of functional imaging to a greater or lesser extent. For other modalities, functional imaging techniques are currently in use either clinically or in the research setting. Examples include diffusion-weighted MR imaging (stroke), MR spectroscopy (mainly research), dynamic-contrast enhanced (DCE) MRI (breast cancer). Most of these newer MR techniques, along with the nuclear medicine techniques have a relatively poor anatomical resolution. Indeed, no modality is perfect; each brings its own advantages and disadvantages, thus the simultaneous use of more than one modality is appealing in that it may overcome the disadvantages of each individual technique. A successful example of multi-modality imaging in current use is that of PET-CT, which produces high resolution anatomical detail through CT, and provides functional information via PET. A further advance in this area may be in the development of multi-modal imaging probes that can be detected by more than one technique.

Another potential means of providing functional imaging is by the use of 'smart' (targeted) contrast agents which can bind specifically to a given target. Such agents exploit factors that are unique to, or preferentially expressed / over-expressed by the target. An example includes exploitation of the 'leakiness' of tumour vessels: tumours undergo neo-angiogenesis in order to sustain growth, however, these new vessels are disorganised and 'leaky'. Larger size imaging agents will preferentially leak through the tumour vasculature but not normal endothelia, thus preferentially enhancing tumours (e.g. DCE-MRI). More specific targeting can be achieved via monoclonal antibodies, or genetically modified fragments on the surface of the contrast agent probe. More important, in terms of tumour response to treatment is the presence of viable cells, potentially future techniques could combine specific tumour targeting through ligands, with subsequent exploitation of factors present only in viable cells (e.g. pH level).

A further advance may lie with the development of new imaging techniques. An example is terahertz radiation ('T-rays'), which does not involve ionising radiation, but can only penetrate a few millimetres into the skin; this is currently being developed for airline security. A further example is that of optical imaging, although imaging is limited by the depth penetration and the presence of white light, there may well be potential for use as an adjunct to endoscopic techniques. Targeted optical probes can be injected intravenously, endoscopes could be then adapted to detect and resolve the relevant fluoroscopic spectrum.

REFERENCE

1   Brenner DJ, Hall EJ. Computed tomography – an increasing source of radiation exposure. *NEJM*. 2007; **357(22)**: 2277–84.

Chapter 4
Objective structured clinical examination (OSCE)

QUESTIONS

1   A patient presents with wrist pain after falling on their outstretched hand. A wrist X-ray is performed.

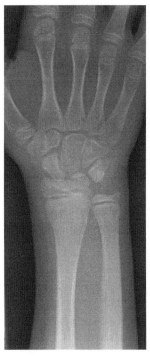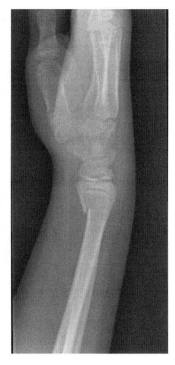

a   Describe the findings.
b   What is the approximate age of this patient?
c   Do you know of any fracture types that are particularly common for patients in this age-group?

2   A 31-year-old man presents to A&E acutely short of breath. A chest X-ray is performed.

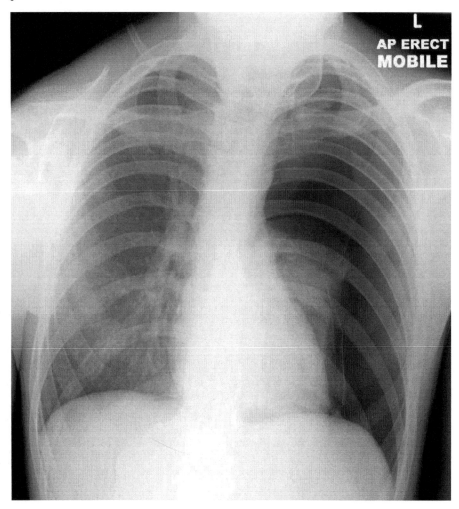

a   What does the CXR show?
b   What causes of this condition do you know?
c   What additional signs would indicate a medical emergency necessitating immediate management?

3 A 67-year-old woman presents with gradually increasing pain in the left knee.

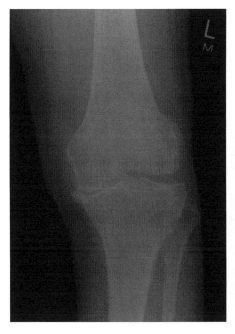 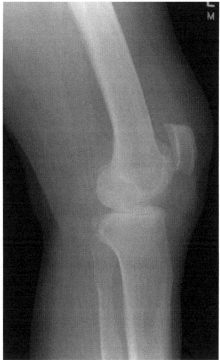

a Describe the findings.
b What is the diagnosis?
c What underlying causes do you know of?

4

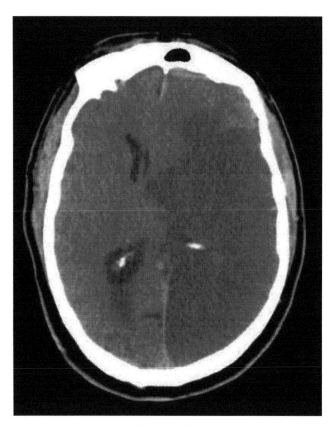

a   What examination has been performed?
b   What is the main finding?
c   What is the underlying diagnosis and how is the patient likely to have presented?

5   A 73-year-old woman presents with left hip pain having fallen. X-rays are performed.

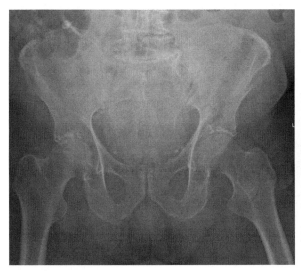 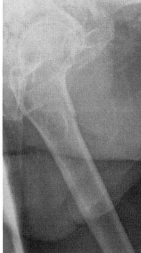

a   Describe the findings.
b   What is the treatment?
c   How does the exact location of the abnormality affect the treatment?

6   A 67-year old woman presents with dyspnoea.

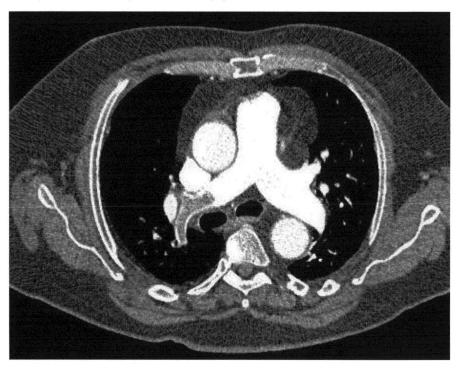

a   What examination is this?
b   What is the main finding?
c   What other radiological test could be used for diagnosis?

7   An adult patient presents with a chronic cough.

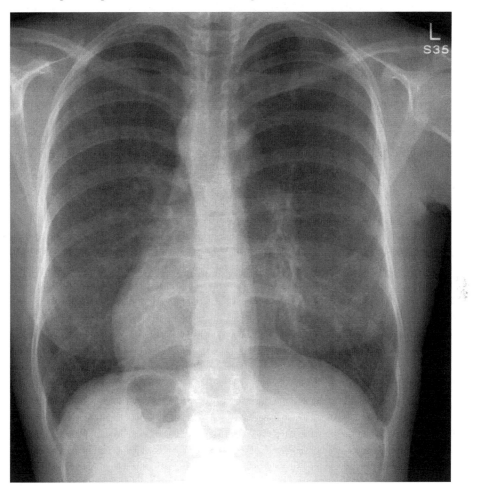

a   Describe the findings.
b   What are the possible causes?
c   What associations do you know of?

8   An 8-year-old boy presents with a limp. The following radiograph is obtained.

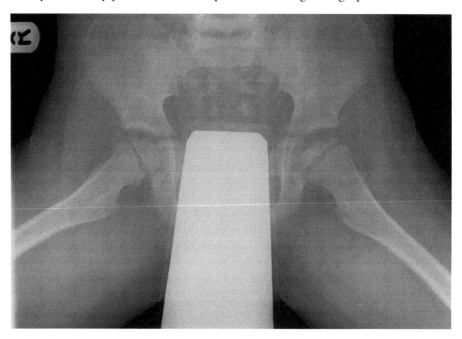

a   What view has been performed?
b   What is the main abnormality?
c   What other conditions should be considered when evaluating a limping child?

9   A 62-year-old man presents with a long history of shortness of breath which has been gradually increasing. A chest X-ray is performed.

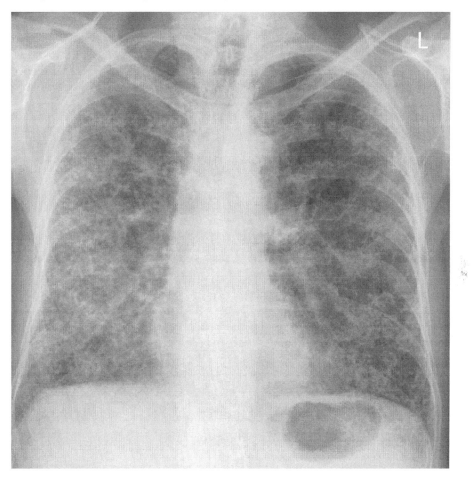

a   Describe the findings.
b   Give three possible underlying causes for these appearances.
c   What are the next steps in the diagnostic work-up?

10

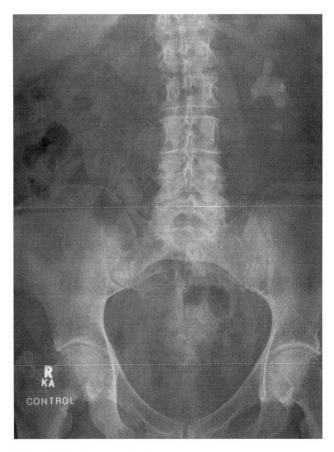

a   What is the abnormality?
b   What type of examination is this image taken from?
c   Which factors predispose to this condition?

11 A 30-year-old man falls on his right elbow.

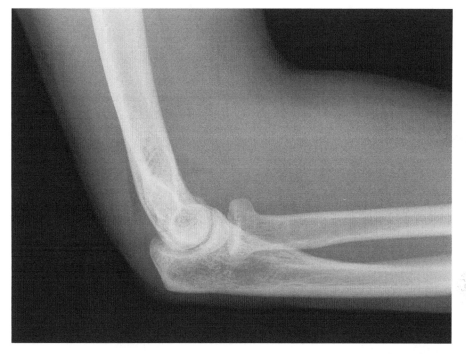

a   What radiological signs are demonstrated?
b   What associated fracture is present?
c   How is this injury managed?

12 A 58-year-old patient presents with a first seizure. A contrast-enhanced CT study is performed.

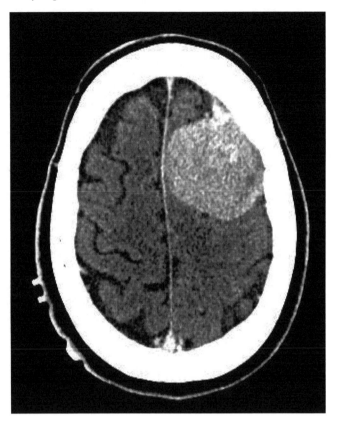

a   What is the main finding?
b   What is the likely diagnosis and how can it be confirmed?
c   Is this likely to be intra or extra-axial?

13 A 22-year-old man presents complaining of chronic foot pain.

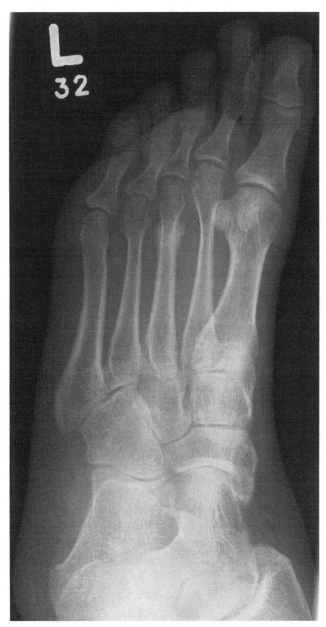

a   Describe the radiological abnormality.
b   What is the diagnosis?
c   Describe typical presentations of this condition.

14 A 46-year-old man presents with general lethargy, and mild shortness of breath on exertion. There is no smoking history. A CXR is performed.

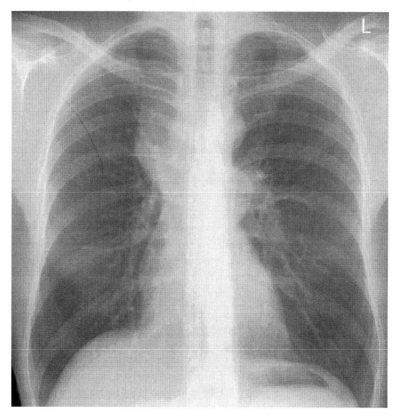

a   Describe the findings.
b   Give two possible underlying causes for these appearances?
c   How can the diagnosis be confirmed?

15

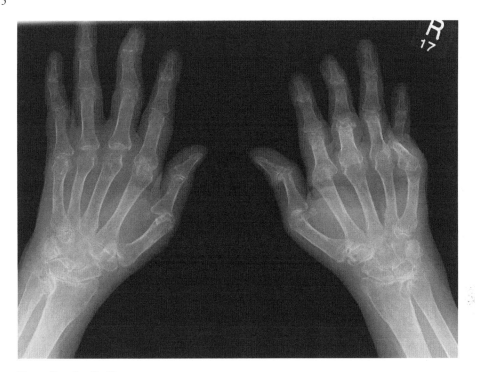

a   Describe the findings.
b   What is the likely underlying diagnosis?
c   What extra-articular features may be associated?

16   A patient presents with acute abdominal pain. An AXR is performed.

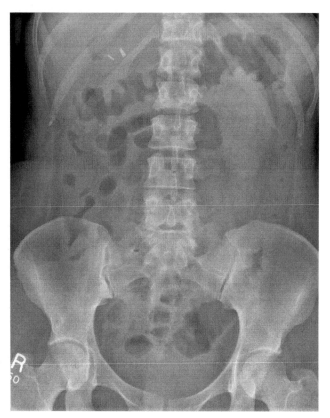

a   Describe the findings.
b   List three possible causes.
c   How could this be further investigated?

17   A 72-year-old patient presents to her GP with a long history of dysphagia.

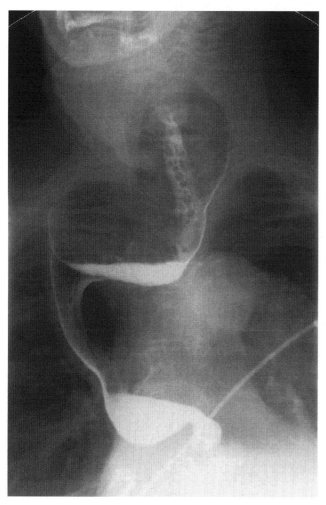

a   What investigation has been performed?
b   What is the likely diagnosis?
c   What other investigations would be appropriate?

18 A 28-year-old, 24/40 weeks pregnant, woman presents with shortness of breath. A number of investigations are performed.

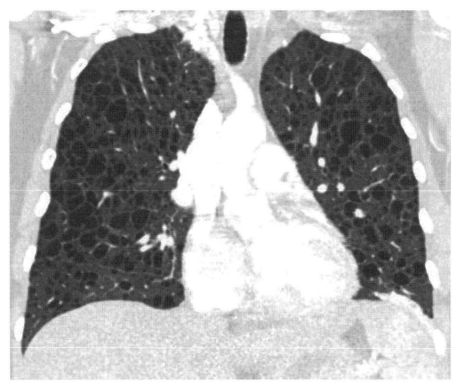

a What imaging test is shown?
b Describe the findings.
c What is the differential diagnosis?
d What complications can arise?

19 A 56-year-old woman presents with gradually increasing pain in the right foot. An X-ray is performed.

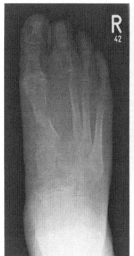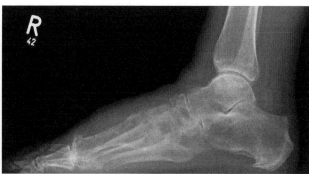

a   Describe the findings.
b   What is the likely cause of these appearances?
c   List two possible underlying diagnoses.

20 A patient presents with increasing cough, shortness of breath and scanty haemoptysis. A CXR is performed.

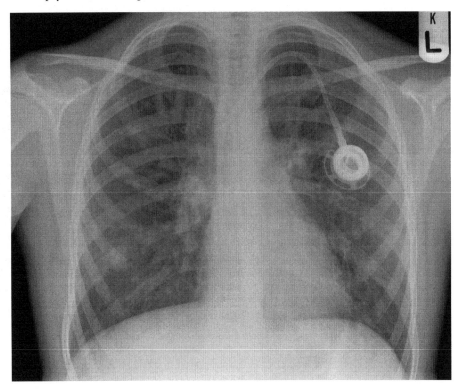

a   Describe the findings.
b   What is the likely diagnosis?
c   Are there signs of infection? If so what organism would you expect?

21 A 32-year-old man presents to his GP with long-standing back pain, which has been gradually increasing. X-rays of the lumbo-sacral spine are requested.

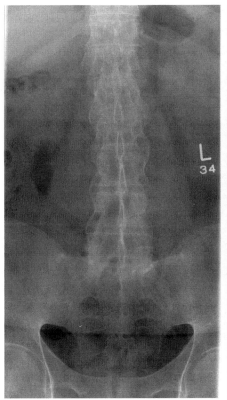 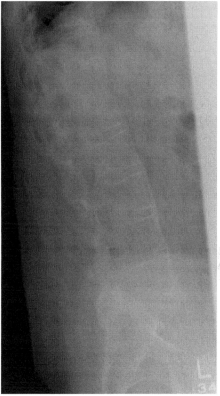

a   Describe the findings.
b   What is likely diagnosis?
c   What associations of this disease do you know?

22 A 10-month-old baby is noted to be short in height for her age. On examination her GP notes a bilateral varus deformity of the knees and requests X-rays.

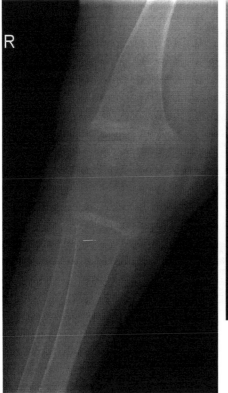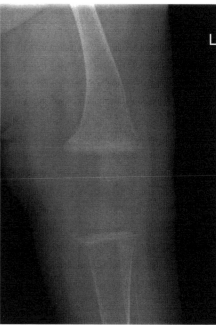

a   Describe the findings.
b   What is the likely diagnosis?
c   What risk factors do you know of?

23

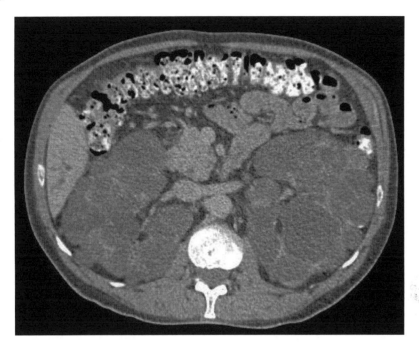

a What examination has been performed?
b Describe the findings.
c What is the likely diagnosis?
d What associations do you know of?

24   You are asked to review a CXR. The request card simply states 'Increased shortness of breath'.

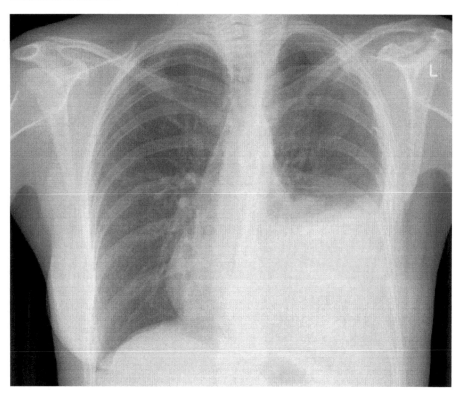

a   What are the main findings?
b   What is the unifying diagnosis?
c   Give three possible causes for the main thoracic finding?

25 A man presents to the emergency department having been punched in the face. He has the following facial radiograph.

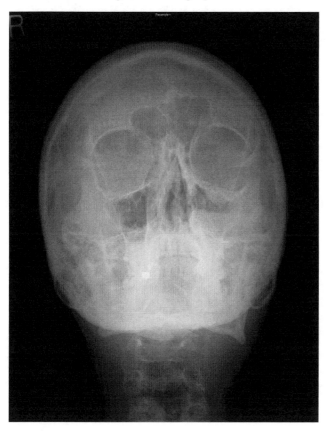

a   Describe the findings.
b   What supporting (non-bony) evidence is there to suggest a fracture?
c   Name this pattern of injury.

26

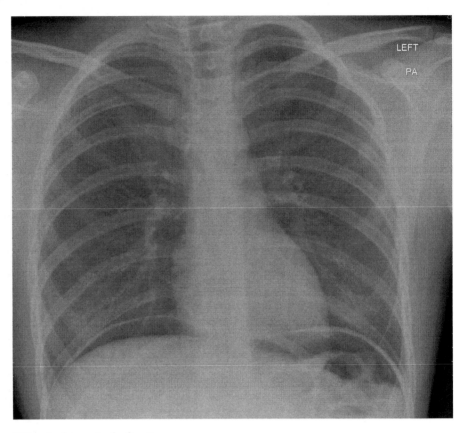

a   What is the main finding?
b   What other radiological investigations are appropriate?
c   List three possible causes.

27

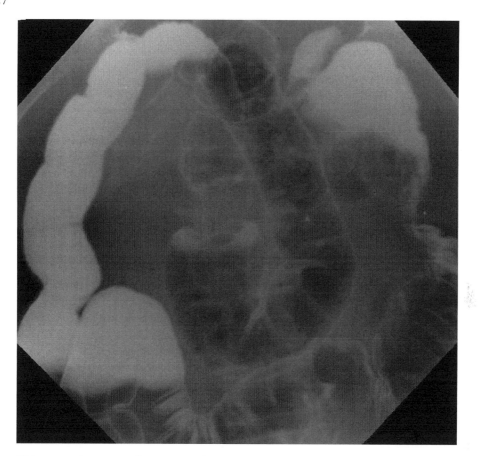

a   What examination is this image taken from?
b   Describe the abnormality.
c   What is the diagnosis?

28

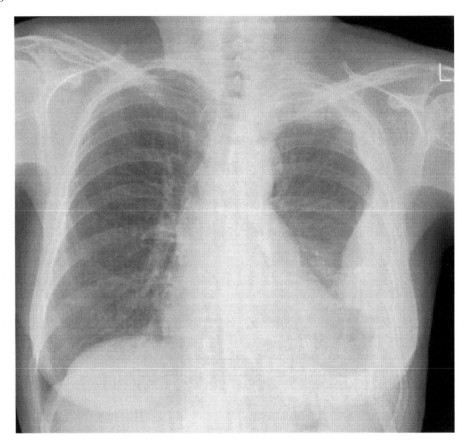

a   Describe the findings.
b   What is the likely diagnosis?
c   What risk factors do you know of for this condition?

29 A 30-year-old man presents to A&E with wrist pain after a fall. On examination
    he is found to be tender in the anatomical snuff box. X-rays are performed.

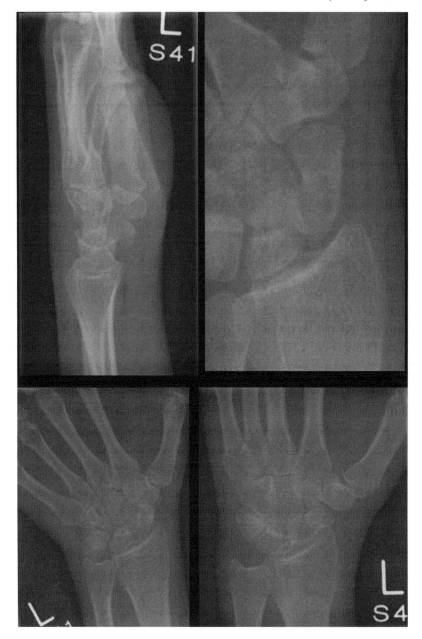

a   Are these images normal or abnormal?
b   What is the next most appropriate course of action with regards to imaging?
c   What is the clinical concern with this type of injury?

30 A 47-year-old previously fit and well woman presents with episodes of epistaxis and haemoptysis. Of note on examination there are several areas of telangiectasia on the patient's tongue. A CXR is performed.

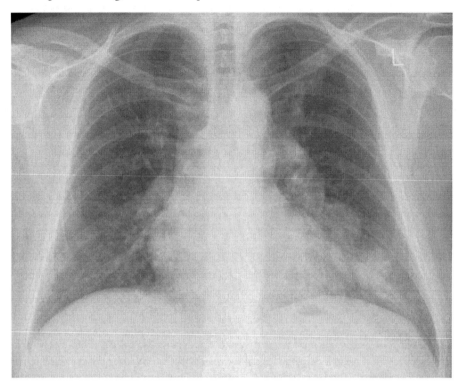

a   Describe the findings.
b   What is the likely underlying diagnosis?
c   Do you know of any possible associated complications?
d   What do you think the treatment options are?

ANSWERS

1

a   The film shows a greenstick type fracture of the distal radius, with a degree of volar angulation apparent on the lateral view. The fracture is seen but is harder to appreciate on the AP view, but clearly demonstrated on the lateral view, emphasising the fact that at least two views are necessary to assess a fracture.

b   The patient's age is 10 years. The key finding is that the epiphyses are yet to fuse, which should be appreciated by the candidate. An age range of 8–16 should be accepted by the examiner.

c   Children's bones are more likely to bend and bow ('plastic bowing fractures') than adult bones, which typically fracture all the way through. As a result there may simply be a 'buckling' of the cortex (buckle fracture), or a break of only one cortex (greenstick fracture). Paediatric fractures which involve the growth plate are classified by the 'Salter-Harris' system and are important because inadequate treatment will affect growth and may result in limb length discrepancy. Below is an example of a Salter-Harris type 2 fracture of the base of the proximal phalanx of the thumb involving the growth plate; a detailed understanding of the subtypes would not be expected.

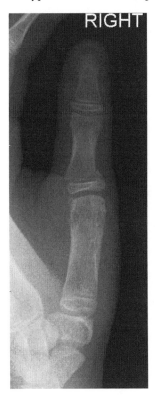

Further reading

*   Raby N, Berman LH, De Lacey G, editors. *Accident & Emergency Radiology*. 2nd ed. London: Elsevier, Saunders; 2005: 306–12.

2

a   There is a left-sided pneumothorax, with almost complete collapse of the
     entire left lung. The initial clue is the difference in density with marked
     hypertranslucency of the left hemithorax compared to the right. There are no
     lung markings present in the periphery of the left hemithorax, and the lung edge
     is clearly seen medially.

b   Trauma is a common cause, from either direct penetrating injuries, or from
     broken ribs. Secondary causes can be idiopathic due to rupture of pulmonary
     'blebs', or due to underlying lung disorders – examples include cystic fibrosis,
     Langerhans cell histiocytosis and lymphangioleiomyomatosis, rupture of bullae
     in COPD, or osteosarcoma metastases. Iatrogenic causes are also possible, for
     example due to positive pressure ventilation, central venous line insertion or
     failed pleural tap.

c   The presence of a 'tension' pneumothorax is a medical emergency necessitating
     immediate treatment. A tension pneumothorax occurs when a one-way valve
     ('ball-valve') occurs at the point of rupture in the lung, air is trapped within the
     pleural cavity and is not released, eventually pressure builds up and compression
     of the heart can result, compromising cardiac output. Clinical signs include:
     signs of pneumothorax (reduced air entry on the affected side, hyper-resonance
     to percussion, etc.), tracheal deviation away from the affected side, and jugular
     venous distension. In theory such cases should be apparent and treatment
     instigated immediately on a clinical basis, before a chest X-ray is performed. The
     CXR signs reflect the clinical findings and include: presence of a pneumothorax,
     and tracheal and mediastinal shift away from the affected side (see image below).
     Treatment is by inserting a 14G needle into the second intercostal space in
     the mid-clavicular line, releasing the pressure and converting the tension into
     a 'simple' pneumothorax, which can subsequently be treated by chest drain
     placement.

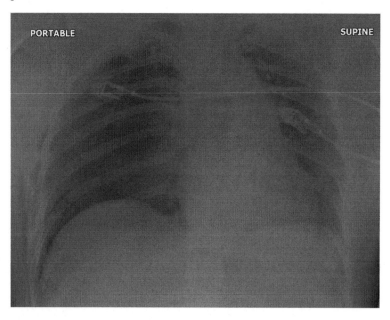

3

a   There is marked loss of joint space within the medial compartment of the knee, with associated varus deformity. This is subchondral sclerosis most marked in the medial tibia. There are osteophytes seen medial to the tibia and within the patella.

b   The findings are those of osteoarthritis. Other plain film findings include subchondral bone cysts.

c   Osetoarthritis can be primary due to degenerative change with age ('wear and tear'). Secondary causes of osteoarthritis include: trauma, inflammatory arthropathies (RhA, gout, pseudogout), metabolic disorders (hemochromatosis, Wilson's disease), septic arthritis, congenital bone / joint problems (causing differences in weight through the joint), recurrent haemarthrosis (particularly secondary to haemophilia), or neuropathy.

4

a   This is an unenhanced CT examination of the head. The high density (white) bones of the cranium make this easy to differentiate from MRI.

b   There is widespread low attenuation within the left hemisphere with associated midline shift to the right. Midline shift is best assessed by drawing a vertical line centrally and assessing displacement of structures (in this case the frontal horns of the lateral ventricles), see image below. Left and right can be confusing to some, but the convention is to always display axial images as if looking up from below, thus the left side of the patient is always the right-hand side of the image.

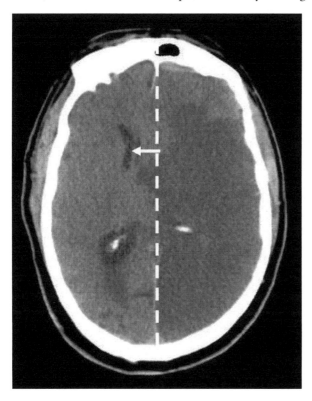

c   The appearances are due to a large ischaemic stroke in the region of the left middle cerebral artery. Given the size of the territory involved, the patient is likely to have presented with significant symptoms: right-sided hemiplegia (paralysis) or hemiparesis ('weakness') and right facial weakness. Speech is also likely to be affected as the left hemisphere is dominant in the majority (90–95% of right-handed and 65–75% of left-handed individuals); loss of consciousness is less likely than with haemorrhagic stroke.

5

a   There is an intertrochanteric fracture of the left neck of femur.

b   These injuries are almost always managed surgically with internal fixation.

c   The type of surgical treatment depends on the location of the fracture in relation to the capsule of the hip joint. If the fracture is extracapsular then internal fixation of the neck of femur using either a dynamic hip screw (DHS) or internal medullary hip screw with preservation of the femoral head can be performed (*see* below). If the fracture is intracapsular then the blood supply to the femoral head is more likely to be compromised, with a high risk of avascular necrosis, therefore the femoral head must be replaced with a prosthesis.

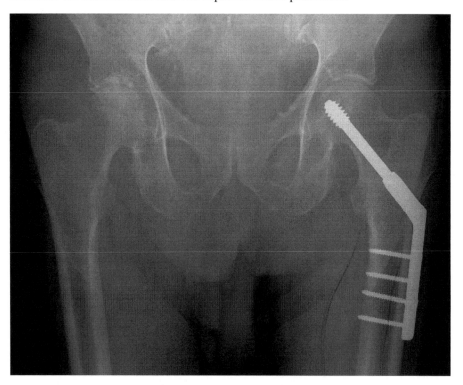

6

a   This is a CT-pulmonary angiogram (CTPA) examination. Contrast medium is seen clearly within the main pulmonary artery.

b   There is a large filling defect within the right main pulmonary artery and extending into the two branches shown (compare this to the normal contrast filled left pulmonary artery). The diagnosis is that of pulmonary embolism.

c   Chest X-ray signs of pulmonary emboli are often non-specific: pleural effusion, atelectasis, enlarged pulmonary arteries; CXR alone cannot confirm the diagnosis. More suggestive signs include pleurally based, wedge shaped opacities, and decreased pulmonary vascularity (Westermark's sign; an area of focal oligaemia). V/Q scans can be used for diagnosis if the chest X-ray is normal.

7

a   There is dextrocardia. In addition, the gastric bubble is seen under the right hemidiaphragm and the left hemidiaphragm is higher than the right, establishing the diagnosis of situs inversus. Note that the 'left' site marker is correctly positioned. Always check the markers; an examiner may deliberately pass such a hard copy film 'backwards' to the candidate to try and catch them out. CT of the upper abdomen in the same patient (below) confirms the abdominal situs inversus, with the liver on the left side of the abdomen and the spleen and stomach on the right. Another abnormality in the CXR is the prominence of the bronchi, with bronchial wall thickening best seen adjacent to the 'left' heart border, consistent with bronchiectasis.

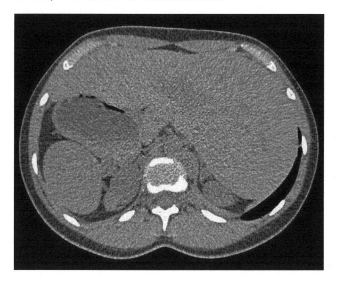

b   The prevalence of situs inversus is approximately 0.01%. There is an increased prevalence of congenital heart disease (5–10%), individuals otherwise have a normal life expectancy. Situs inversus can occur spontaneously, or be inherited in an autosomal recessive or X-linked manner. Approximately 25% of people with situs inversus have Kartagener's syndrome (also known as primary ciliary dyskinesia), as in this case, as confirmed by the presence of bronchiectasis.

c   Kartagener's syndrome is characterised by the triad of situs inversus, chronic sinusitis, and bronchiectasis, all secondary to poor ciliary function. The bronchiectasis suggested at CXR, is confirmed in this patient's chest CT (*see* below). There is also an association with subfertility (females) or infertility (males), otitis media, impaired sense of smell and reduced hearing.

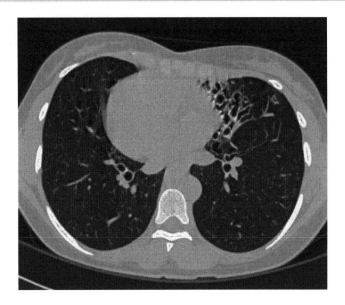

8

a   This is a 'frog-leg' lateral view performed with the child lying down with external rotation and flexion of the hip joints and flexion of the knee joint.

b   The main abnormality is flattening, deformity and segmentation of the left femoral epiphysis. The features are those of Perthe's disease. Perthe's disease typically affects children in the 4–8 year age group, this is an idiopathic condition that causes avascular necrosis of the femoral epiphysis. Other radiological features include joint space widening, sclerosis of the femoral epiphysis and subchondral cyst formation.

c   The main differentials when considering a limping child include septic arthritis, transient synovitis, Perthe's disease, and slipped upper femoral epiphysis. Septic arthritis most commonly presents before the age of three years. Hip ultrasound may demonstrate an effusion, however plain films are generally rather insensitive. Transient synovitis is a benign self-limiting condition considered to be of viral aetiology which affects children in the 4–10 year age group and which resolves over 48–72 hours. SUFE affects an older age group than Perthe's (typically overweight adolescents) and is bilateral in 20% of cases. The femoral epiphysis undergoes posterior-medial slip and is best appreciated on the frog-leg view. Treatment is surgical with insertion of pins to hold the epiphysis in the correct position.

9

a   There is bilateral, diffuse reticulo-nodular opacification with no apparent areas of sparing. There is distortion of the cardiac outline and the hemidiaphragms. The findings are consistent with diffuse interstitial lung fibrosis.

b   There are numerous causes of pulmonary fibrosis, it is easiest to break these down into subgroups:

    •   Idiopathic: sarcoid, UIP, NSIP, or desquamative interstitial pneumonitis (DIP).

- Inhaled substances: silicosis, asbestosis, berylliosis.
- Infective: TB, PCP, RSV.
- Connective tissue disorders: scleroderma, SLE, RhA.
- Drug induced: chemotherapy agents, antiarrhythmics.
- Malignancy: lymphangitic carcinomatosis.

c   The work-up is a combination of radiological, clinical and pathological findings to reach the underlying diagnosis. Pulmonary function tests should be performed, these will show a restrictive pattern if there is fibrosis. In terms of radiology the next step would be high-resolution CT (HRCT) of the chest. CT findings include ground-glass opacification, bronchiectasis, and architectural distortion, and eventually honeycombing when there is established fibrosis. The distribution may also give clues to the diagnosis, for instance a basal and peripheral (subpleural) distribution is consistent with a diagnosis of usual interstitial fibrosis (UIP).

10
a   There is a 'staghorn' calculus within the left kidney.
b   This is the control film (i.e. the initial pre-contrast image) from an IVU examination (as evidenced by the label in the bottom left corner of the image). This information enables one to be certain that this is truly a calculus rather than contrast medium filling the pelvicalyceal system.
c   With solitary episodes of small calculi a specific cause is often not identified. Generally, the causes of calculi can broadly be divided into:

- Infection – e.g. Proteus spp. (particularly cause staghorn calculi).
- Stasis – due to renal tract obstruction and congenital abnormalities.
- Metabolic – due to hyperparathyroidism, hypercalciuria, gout or polycythemia.

11
a   There is a posterior fat pad sign present, a lucent line behind the distal humerus (which is always an abnormal finding). In addition, there is subtle elevation of the anterior fat pad. These are signs of a joint effusion.
b   Careful scrutiny demonstrates a radial head fracture. In the presence of a positive fat sign in this age group, the radial head should be carefully examined. On occasions a fracture line may not be evident, nevertheless, these patients are still treated as presumed, occult radial head fractures (assuming no other obvious fracture).
c   Treatment depends on the severity of the injury and ranges from conservative management with a collar and cuff (most likely in this case), through to operative intervention involving excision +/– replacement of the radial head.

12
a   There is a well-circumscribed high attenuation lesion with the left frontal region. There is contrast-enhancement within the lesion and focal areas of high attenuation anteriorly which suggest calcification. There is also the suggestion of a 'dural tail' seen at the anterior aspect of the lesion.

b   The imaging features are classic for a meningioma, the likely 'dural tail', which is better characterised at MRI, is further evidence of this diagnosis (seen in up to 70%). Imaging findings may be highly suggestive of the diagnosis, a lumbar puncture may show elevated CSF protein, but neurosurgical biopsy is definitive for diagnosis.

c   Meningiomas arise from the arachnoidal cells and are thus extra-axial. Common locations include the fronto-parietal region, the falx, the cerebello-pontine angle, the olfactory groove, and the sphenoid ridge. They are typically slow growing and are often found incidentally.

13

a   There is periosteal reaction and callus formation around the neck of the third metatarsal.

b   The diagnosis is a stress or 'overuse' fracture.

c   Typical presentations are those where there is a history of chronic repetitive strain on the bone. These injuries are commonly seen in soldiers (originally described as 'march' fractures) and runners (of all abilities!).

14

a   There is a mass within the right hemithorax, just above the right hilum. This forms obtuse angles with the mediastinum, implying that it originates from here, rather than the lung. The superior aspect of the right heart border is lost, but the hilar structures are seen clearly (thus it is not in the middle mediastinum) and the mass does not extend above the right clavicle (posterior mediastinal masses can do this, anterior ones cannot). The mass is therefore located within the anterior mediastinum.

b   The differential diagnosis for an anterior mediastinal mass is the '4 Ts': thymoma, teratoma (germ cell tumours), thyroid, and 'terrible' lymph nodes (often due to lymphoma). Thymoma is the commonest primary tumour of the anterior mediastinal in adults (20%), but is rarely seen in children.

c   A lateral CXR may help confirm the anterior location of the mass. A staging CT of the chest will give additional information, including local invasion and distant spread, however, tissue is required for diagnosis. Biopsy can be performed at mediastinoscopy, or, if accessible, tissue can be obtained transbronchially at bronchoscopy or percutaneously by CT-guidance.

15

a   There is a bilateral, predominantly symmetrical deforming arthropathy of the hands. There is hyperextension of the PIP joints and hyperflexion of the DIP joints of the third and the fifth digits, resulting in 'swan neck' deformities, and there is a 'Z-shaped' deformity of the thumbs, more marked on the right. There is involvement of the MCP joints, slight ulna deviation of the wrist joint, and erosion of the right ulna styloid process. There is also noted to be periarticular osteopenia.

b   The diagnosis is rheumatoid arthritis. The differential diagnosis is that of rheumatoid-like psoriatic arthritis. The listed features are all those of RhA, further features include Boutonniere deformity (PIP joint hyperflexion, with DIP joint hyperextension).

c   Extra-articular features are present in about 15–25% of patients. Examples include lung fibrosis, skin nodules, pleural effusion, pericarditis, vasculitis, skin manifestations (including livedo reticularis, pyoderma gangrenosum, erythema nodosum), nephropathy, amyloidosis, peripheral neuropathy, episcleritis, and osteoporosis.

16

a   There is oedematous bowel with thickening of the transverse colon wall, with associated thumb-printing. There is also marked oedematous thickening of the wall of the descending colon, with associated collapse of the bowel. There is no evidence of obstruction and no evidence of perforation.

b   The findings are those of colitis, causes include:
   •   Ischaemic colitis.
   •   Inflammatory colitis (Crohn's disease / ulcerative colitis).
   •   Pseudomembranous colitis (e.g. due to Clostridium difficile).
   •   Other causes of infective colitis: amoebic, schistosomiasis.
   •   haemolytic uraemic syndrome in children.
   •   Lymphomatous infiltration.
   •   Rare causes: post-radiotherapy, post-barium enema examination, metastases.

c   Simple test such as stool cultures, FBC, inflammatory markers and serology should be initially performed. Depending on the clinical context, or concern, CT may be appropriate, e.g. looking for evidence of ischaemic colitis, or intra-abdominal infective collections. However, direct visualisation by rigid / flexi-sigmoidoscopy or colonoscopy is preferred, and biopsies can also be taken if required.

17

a   This is a barium swallow study. The patient is asked to drink a contrast agent (usually barium) and under fluoroscopy screening, multiple images are taken from different positions. The study gives information on oesophageal motility and structural abnormalities within the oesophagus.

b   The likely diagnosis is primary (idiopathic) achalasia. In this condition, there is oesophageal dysmotility and a failure of relaxation of the lower oesophageal sphincter (LES). This produces increased pressure at the LES and a tight tapering at the GOJ, resulting in a 'bird's beak' or 'rat's tail' appearance. There is a dilated, patulous oesophagus proximal to this. Other, 'secondary' causes of achalasia include diabetes mellitus / neuropathy, Chagas disease, and scleroderma. The lateral wall of the dilated oesophagus may be visible on the CXR (*see* below), and may cause confusion to the un-trained eye. On a barium swallow there is often significant hold-up of barium at the GOJ, which subsequently passes easily on swallowing hot water (*see* examples below from a different patient).

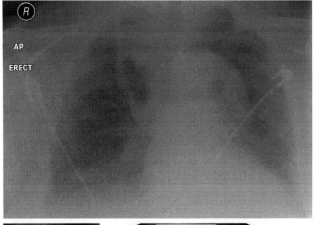

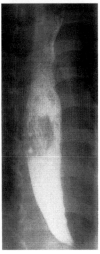
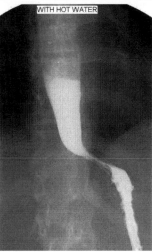

c   Oesophageal manommetry tests can confirm the diagnosis. OGD is useful to rule-out a malignant stricture in cases of doubt, biopsies will show hypertrophied muscle, with absence of myenteric plexus cells. An autoimmune screen looking for evidence of secondary causes of achalasia (e.g. scleroderma) may be appropriate. Treatment can be by dilatation at OGD, direct injection of muscle relaxants (botulinum toxin), or more definitively by myomotomy (Heller procedure).

18

a   This is a CT chest examination. This has been reformatted and viewed in the coronal plane, on lung window settings. If the axial CT is acquired with a narrow slice thickness (≤ 2 mm), reconstruction can easily be performed in the coronal or sagittal planes.

b   There are multiple, small thin-walled cystic lesions throughout both lungs. The background lung parenchyma has a 'ground-glass' appearance. There is no pneumothorax. An axial CT slice from the same series is shown below for reference.

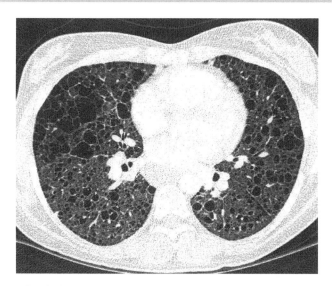

c   The differential diagnosis is that of cystic lung disease in adults; by definition
     lung cysts at CT have a wall ≤ 2 mm. The differential in younger patients is
     between lymphangioleiomyomatosis (LAM) and Langerhans cell histiocytosis
     (LCH). LAM has similar size cysts with no zonal preference, is associated
     with chylous pleural effusions, is seen in female patients, and is associated
     with tuberous sclerosis. LCH predominantly affects the upper zones in young,
     male smokers, has associated nodules, bizarre shaped cysts, and spares the
     medial aspects of the middle and lingular lobes. Other causes include bullous
     emphysema, cystic bronchiectasis, and pneumatocoeles. In this young female
     patient, with known tuberous sclerosis, the diagnosis was LAM.

d   Rupture of a cyst can lead to pneumothorax: see CXR below in the same patient six
     weeks later; also note the hyperinflation caused by the condition. Obstructive type
     respiratory compromise can result. LAM specifically may cause chylothorax due to
     thickening of the lymphatics, also pulmonary oedema or haemorrhage; symptoms
     often worsen with use of the OCP or during pregnancy (as with this patient).

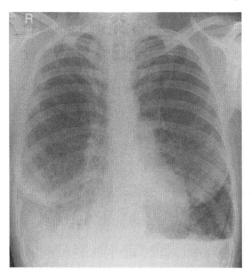

19

a There is complete absence of the second metatarsal, there is also a lytic lesion within the base of the first metatarsal medially. The joint spaces are relatively well preserved.

b The complete absence of a second metatarsal implies an aggressive lesion; this could be due to a primary bone tumour, metastases, or infection. However, the additional lytic lesion in the first metatarsal makes metastases the far more likely diagnosis.

c In this female patient, the underlying diagnosis was breast cancer. Other common causes of lytic bone metastases include renal cell carcinoma and lung cancer.

20

a This is a frontal chest radiograph in a teenage patient, where the right humeral epiphysis is noted to be unfused. There is a tunnelled left subclavian port-a-cath with its tip appropriately sited in the right atrium. There is dilation of the upper lobe bronchi, with wall thickening, consistent with bronchiectasis. Within both upper zones there are tubular opacities radiating from the hilum to the periphery, with a classic 'finger-in-glove' appearance due to mucus plugging in the airways. There is a patch of consolidation in the right lower zone. There is no pneumothorax.

b This is a young patient with evidence of bronchiectasis with upper lobe predominance and mucoid impaction ('finger-in-glove opacity'), and with a tunnelled line; the diagnosis is cystic fibrosis. As a general rule, tunnelled lines will be present for i.v. access in order to administer either long-term courses of antibiotics or chemotherapy. Another clue to cystic fibrosis would be the presence of rib fractures due to excessive coughing (not seen in this case).

c The mucoid impaction and patch of consolidation in the RLZ imply recent infection. 'Finger-in-glove' opacification is classsically described in aspergillus infection (allergic bronchopulmonary aspergillosis (ABPA)), which is a common infective organism in CF. CF patients of this age are also prone to the following chest infections: mycobacterium avium complex, pseudomonas aeruginosa, and burkholderia cepacia.

21

a On the AP film there is marked sclerosis and fusion of the sacroiliac joints, there is also sclerosis and apparent fusion of the spinous processes. The lateral film shows sclerosis of the endplates and calcification of the anterior spinal ligaments, forming a 'bony bridge' between the vertebral bodies.

b The findings are those of ankylosing spondylitis. AS is a chronic, inflammatory sero-negative arthritis. The main pathology is enthesitis (inflammation of the tendons as they insert into bone). It has a predilection for the axial skeleton, and particularly affects the sacroiliac and spinal facet joints, eventually leading to spinal fusion (bamboo spine). Note the fusion of the cervical facet joints in the example below:

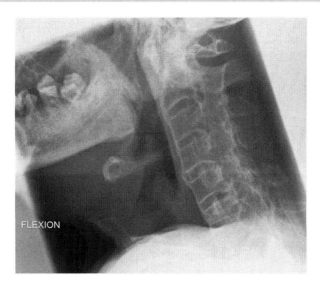

FLEXION

c   Approximately 90% of patients with ankylosing spondylitis are HLA-B27 positive. Extra-articular associations include iridocyclitis / uveitis, aortitis, and upper zone lung fibrosis.

22

a   There is fraying and splaying of the metaphyses, with the suggestion of growth plate widening, and early 'cupping' of the epiphyses. Although not fully imaged, there is apparent bowing of the left femur. Overall there is poor mineralisation of the bones imaged.

b   The findings are those of Rickets. Other X-ray features include periosteal reaction, cortical spurs seen at right angles to the metaphyses, coarse trabeculation, poor dentition, craniotabes (soft skull), frontal bossing, and rachitic rosary (splaying) of the ribs. Blood tests typically show a low calcium, low phosphate and raised alkaline phosphatase. The condition is analogous to osteomalacia in adults (with a fused skeleton).

c   Risk factors include vitamin D deficiency due to lack of sunlight exposure. Dietary deficiency of vitamin D or calcium can also be a cause (poor nutrition, pancreatitis, malabsorption syndromes). Liver or renal impairment is also a risk factor (defective conversion of vitamin D subunits).

23

a   This is a CT examination of the abdomen following the administration of oral and intravenous contrast media. Oral contrast is seen within the transverse colon anteriorly.

b   There is bilateral enlargement and cystic replacement of the renal tissue. There is also the suggestion of cystic change in the inferior tip of the right lobe of the liver seen on this slice.

c   The diagnosis is adult (autosomal dominant) polycystic kidney disease. The differential is of bilateral cystic renal disease, which includes autosomal recessive polycystic kidney disease (cysts tend to be small), VHL (tend to be less cysts, you would expect additional solid renal lesions; pancreatic cysts may also be seen), tuberous sclerosis, or bilateral simple renal cyst (unlikely to be so numerous).

d   Approximately 50% will develop end-stage renal disease by the age of 60. Hypertension is common and there is an increased incidence of UTIs and renal stones. There is also an association with berry aneurysms, aortic root dilation and mitral and aortic valvular dysfunction. Patients may present with hypertension, pain / haematuria from cyst rupture, renal failure, or screening in family relatives (usually by US in early adulthood).

24

a   There is a large left pleural effusion, with evidence of slight mediastinal shift to the right (the inferior trachea and heart are displaced). In addition there has been a previous left mastectomy, and surgical clips are seen within the left axillary, consistent with a previous axillary lymph node clearance for breast cancer. The left mastectomy is harder to appreciate due to the presence of the pleural effusion, but should still be noted by the candidate; remember the 'soft tissue' review areas.

b   Malignant left pleural effusion secondary to breast cancer. The higher stage of the primary breast cancer is suggested by the previous mastectomy (rather than wide local excision) and the evidence of prior lymph node clearance, which is not undertaken for lower stage disease, or when the sentinel node(s) are negative. In an exam situation any clues on the radiograph should be considered pertinent, the examiner may even state the clichéd words '...*the answer is on the film*'. For example, in the case of dilated cardiomyopathy (DCM) shown below, there is also noted to be a left mastectomy. This is not co-incidental: the patient had premorbidly normal cardiac function; the DCM is secondary to adjuvant anthracycline chemotherapy for her breast cancer. Herceptin™ is also associated with DCM; the risk is significantly increased if the two drugs are used concurrently.

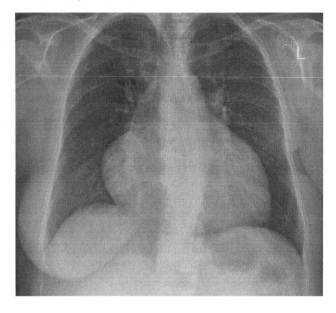

c   There are numerous causes of a pleural effusion, which can be broadly grouped as transudates (protein < 30 g/L) or exudates. Transudative causes include CCF, liver failure, renal failure, and low protein states (e.g. malnutrition, nephrotic syndrome, post-operative). Exudative causes include infection, malignancy (primary or secondary), pulmonary emboli, pancreatitis, and connective tissue disorders (e.g. rheumatoid arthritis).

25
a   There is a fracture of the left zygomatic arch, widening of the zygomatico-frontal suture (diastasis) and a fracture through the body of the zygoma which manifests itself as an inferior orbital rim fracture.
b   There is a fluid level within the left maxillary sinus which is likely to represent haemorrhage (note the normal right maxillary sinus). In addition there is added soft tissue immediately inferior to the orbital rim which represents herniation of some of the orbital contents inferiorly. This is called the 'teardrop' sign and represents a 'blow-out' fracture of the orbit.
c   The combination of these injuries is referred to as a 'tripod' fracture.

26
a   There is air seen under both hemidiaphragms. This is likely to be secondary to a perforated viscus; 'pseudo' pneumoperitoneum can be seen if bowel is interposed between the right hemidiaphragm and the dome of the liver (Chilaiditi syndrome), or if a band of linear atelectasis is seen just superior to the diaphragm.
b   An abdominal X-ray can show free air; the signs are often subtle on a supine film, but this may be useful in showing an underlying cause. The supine film below in the same patient shows a slither of free air in the RUQ, under the liver. An example of a left lateral decubitus AXR (left-side down) in a different patient clearly shows free air above the liver. An abdominal CT can confirm the diagnosis (this study is performed supine, thus free air rises centrally rather than to the hemidiaphragms), this may help to localise the region of perforation pre-operatively.

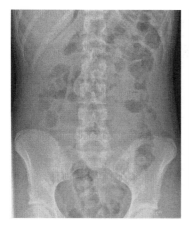
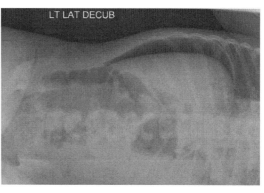

LT LAT DECUB

c Causes include perforation of an abdominal viscus (e.g. secondary to a duodenal ulcer, a gastric ulcer, or a colonic diverticulum), penetrating abdominal trauma, post surgical (laparotomy / lapaoscopy), inflammatory / infective (e.g. appendicitis, cholecystitis, toxic megacolon), or peritoneal dialysis. In this young patient the perforation was secondary to appendicitis.

27
a This is an image from a double contrast barium enema study. Initially contrast medium is instilled rectally, then air is insufflated to allow better delineation of the bowel mucosa by barium. The use of barium enemas for the investigation of suspected colorectal tumours has declined sharply in recent years as the use of first colonoscopy and then CT colonography has become more widespread.
b The major abnormality is an irregular 'apple-core' like stricture within the sigmoid colon.
c The diagnosis is primary colonic carcinoma.

28
a There is lobulated pleural thickening within the left hemithorax. This is most pronounced laterally and there is additional involvement of the mediastinal pleura, with almost complete encasement of the left lung. The apparent lesion in the left apex forms obtuse borders with the chest wall and is likely to represent further pleurally based disease rather than a discrete lesion in the lung parenchyma. There is no associated pleural effusion.
b The diagnosis is mesothelioma. The mesothelium is the epithelial cuboidal cell lining of the serous cavities including the peritoneum, pericardium, and the pleural. Recurrent pleural effusions can be problematic and can be treated with talc-pleuradesis. The work-up includes CT chest. Pleural thickening and plaques are markers of prior asbestos exposure and do not necessarily imply mesothelioma; CT indicators of malignant pleural thickening include: involvement of the mediastinal pleura, nodularity, thickening > 1 cm, and encasement. Diagnosis can be confirmed by tapping any pleural effusion and sending for cytology, or biopsying areas of pleural thickening.
c The risk of mesothelioma is increased 30× by exposure to asbestos, although the condition may not appear until 30 years after the original asbestos exposure. Other risk factors / association are prior radiation therapy, intra-pleural thorotrast (used as a radiological contrast agent until the 1950s), and inhalation of other fibrous silicates (similar to asbestos); there is no proven association between mesothelioma and smoking. There are different types of asbestos fibre, the risk of mesothelioma is as follows: crocidolite (blue) > amosite (brown) > chrysotile (white). Asbestos exposure is also associated with asbestosis, a type of pneumoconosis causing interstitial lung disease.

29
a These images form a 'scaphoid series', in which four views are standard. No scaphoid fracture is demonstrated.
b It is well recognised that scaphoid fractures can be radiologically occult immediately after they occur and therefore follow up is indicated 8–14 days

after the initial injury if no fracture is initially seen, provided the patient remains symptomatic. However, there are a proportion of patients where clinical concern persists (i.e. ongoing pain / tenderness) and the two scaphoid series appear normal. In these cases further imaging with either MRI or bone scintigraphy (depending on the local protocol / availability) is recommended. In this case a bone scintigram demonstrated increased trace uptake in the left scaphoid confirming the fracture, *see* below (note the normal uptake in the right hand for comparison). In nuclear medicine tracer 'site markers' are placed on the right (the dot seen on the far left of the image).

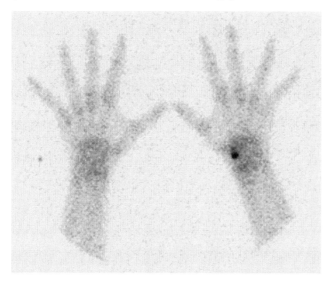

c   The significance of these injuries relates to the blood supply to the scaphoid. The majority of the blood supply enters just distal to the waist and the proximal pole is supplied by retrograde branches from this point. Therefore a proximal pole or proximal waist fracture is associated with a relatively high degree of avascular necrosis of the scaphoid.

30

a   There is a serpiginous structure which runs along the left heart border and appears contiguous with the left pulmonary artery. There are no focal lung nodules, the right pulmonary artery appears of normal calibre, and the heart size is at the upper limit of normal.

b   The diagnosis is a pulmonary arteriovenous malformation (PAVM), the collateral evidence in the vignette points to an underlying diagnosis of hereditary haemorrhagic telangiectasia (HHT; Osler-Weber-Rendu syndrome). This is an abnormal connection between the pulmonary artery and the pulmonary veins, bypassing the capillaries. The contrast-enhanced chest CT in the same patient (*see* below), clearly shows the vascular nature of this abnormality. PAVMs are usually congenital, there is also a strong association with HHT (up to 20% of these patients, often with multiple PAVMs). PAVM can be secondary to trauma, iatrogenic intervention (lung biopsy), liver cirrhosis, or infection.

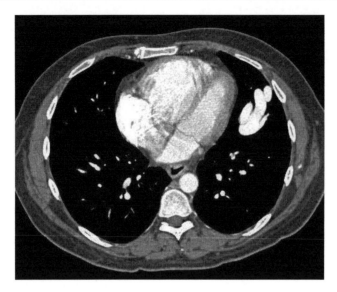

c   The pulmonary capillaries are bypassed, which causes a right to left shunt, this
    can result in CCF, paradoxical emboli, and brain abscesses. There is also a risk of
    massive haemoptysis.
d   The usual treatment is by interventional angiography and embolisation. Coils
    or detachable balloons are used to pack the pulmonary vein and embolise the
    connection. Particulate embolisation material is not used due to the risk of non-
    target embolisation to the systemic circulation / brain. Surgery is considered
    when the AVM is > 1 cm or if the risk of systemic embolisation is considered
    significant.

Chapter 5
Multiple choice questions (MCQs)

QUESTIONS

1 Advantages of MRI imaging of the abdomen over CT abdomen include the following.
  a Faster acquisition time.
  b Better spatial resolution.
  c Fewer contra-indications.
  d Less prone to patient-related artefacts.
  e Lower radiation dose.

2 Ultrasound is indicated for the investigation of the following suspected diagnoses?
  a Cholecystitis.
  b Osteomyelitis.
  c Pancoast tumour.
  d Pyelonephritis.
  e Deep venous thrombosis.

3 A two-year-old child is at high risk for NAI. Which of the following are advantages of bone scintigraphy over skeletal survey?
  a Lower radiation dose.
  b Quicker to perform.
  c More sensitive for fractures.
  d More specific for fractures.
  e Better at demonstrating fractures of different ages.

4 A 16-week pregnant woman presents to A&E with chest pain, the working diagnosis is pulmonary emboli. The following statements are true in this patient.
  a CTPA produces a higher radiation dose to the foetus.
  b A V/Q scan produces a higher radiation dose to the mother.
  c A D-dimer blood test is a useful investigation.
  d Pulmonary angiography is the first line radiological investigation.
  e Bilateral lower limb Doppler US is indicated in the absence of unilateral leg swelling.

5   For which of the following suspected clinical diagnoses would it be appropriate
    to perform an AXR as a first line investigation?
    a   Acute GI bleeding.
    b   Small bowel obstruction.
    c   Chronic pancreatitis.
    d   Appendicitis.
    e   Renal colic.

6   Which of the following conditions occur more frequently in premature rather
    than post-mature neonates?
    a   Birth trauma.
    b   Meconium aspiration.
    c   Necrotising entero-colitis.
    d   Patent ductus arteriosus.
    e   Respiratory distress syndrome.

7   Which of the following features describe an extradural (epidural) haematoma?
    a   Typically crescentic in shape.
    b   Usually due to arterial bleeding.
    c   Commonly associated with non-accidental injury in children.
    d   Commonly associated with skull fractures.
    e   Commonest in the temporal bone region.

8   Which of the following imaging features are more suggestive of a diagnosis of
    Crohn's colitis rather than ulcerative colitis?
    a   Multiple anal fistulae.
    b   Skip lesions.
    c   Toxic megacolon.
    d   Strictures.
    e   Sclerosing cholangitis.

9   Which of the following are known associations of cystic fibrosis?
    a   Gallstones.
    b   Pectus excavatum.
    c   Low sodium concentration in sweat.
    d   Meconium plug syndrome.
    e   Pneumothorax.

10 CT is an excellent method of investigation for which of the following?
    a   Diagnosing gastric carcinoma.
    b   Identifying renal tract stones in a patient with renal colic.
    c   Identifying bladder tumours.
    d   Staging for colorectal cancer.
    e   Evaluating complications of pancreatitis.

11 In most UK hospitals, a radiologist will perform the majority of the following procedures.
a   Endoscopic retrograde cholangiopancreatogram.
b   Coronary angiography.
c   Lower limb angioplasty for peripheral vascular disease.
d   Radiotherapy.
e   Stent placement in SVC obstruction.

12 Regarding gallstones, the following statements are true.
a   Occur in 10–15% of the adult UK population.
b   5x more common in women.
c   Ultrasound is the best radiological investigation.
d   Found in two thirds of patients with pancreatitis.
e   90% of stones are radio-opaque.

13 Regarding the management and radiological assessment of a safe swallow in a patient following a stroke, the following statements are true.
a   Aspiration increases with posterior head tilt.
b   Aspiration is more likely with thick rather than thin fluids.
c   Gastrografin® is the ideal contrast agent.
d   Gastrostomy tubes can only be inserted radiologically.
e   AP views are optimal for assessment.

14 A man presents with shortness of breath. CXR shows a near 'white out' of the right lung with displacement of the mediastinum to the left. The differential diagnosis includes?
a   Mesothelioma.
b   Collapse.
c   Post pneumonectomy.
d   Pleural effusion.
e   Consolidation.

15 Regarding obstetrical ultrasound, which of the following are true?
a   The umbilical cord contains two arteries and one vein.
b   The routine anomaly US scan is performed at 12 weeks.
c   US-guided amniocentesis is performed earlier than chorionic villus sampling.
d   IUGR is most accurately diagnosed by measuring the head circumference to abdominal circumference ratio.
e   The crown-rump length is used in the second trimester.

16 Which of the following conditions will cause the heart to appear falsely enlarged on a chest X-ray?
a   Emphysema.
b   PA film.
c   Patient is rotated.
d   Poor patient inspiration.
e   Supine film.

17   Which of the following statements in relation to fracture descriptions are true?
   a   The direction of displacement is described in relation to the proximal fragment.
   b   Avulsion fractures are caused by tendon or ligaments.
   c   If the skin surface is broken the fracture is described as comminuted.
   d   Pseudoarthrosis describes delayed union between fracture fragments.
   e   If there is separation between fragments this is termed distraction.

18   It is necessary to advise a woman that breast feeding needs to be avoided for a set time period following which of these radiological examinations?
   a   Abdominal X-ray.
   b   CT chest, abdomen, and pelvis.
   c   MRI head.
   d ^{99m}Tc-white blood cell scan.
   e ^{18}FDG-PET scan.

19   Regarding Meckel's diverticulum the following statements are true.
   a   Is a true diverticulum.
   b   Gastric mucosa is present in 95–100%.
   c   Is usually found on the mesenteric border.
   d   Diverticulitis is the commonest presentation.
   e   Nuclear medicine ^{99m}Tc-Pertechnetate studies are the most sensitive for diagnosis.

20   The following are recognised causes of polyhydramnios in pregnancy.
   a   Intrauterine growth retardation.
   b   Oesophageal atresia.
   c   Rhesus incompatibility.
   d   Infantile (autosomal recessive) polycystic kidney disease.
   e   Maternal diabetes.

21   Regarding breast ultrasound, which of the following statements is true?
   a   Can be used as an alternative to mammography for breast cancer screening.
   b   Is used to evaluate non-palpable lesions that have been detected at mammography.
   c   An anechoic lesion is cancer until proven otherwise.
   d   Is the most sensitive method for detecting rupture of silicone breast implants.
   e   US-guided biopsy is preferable over stereotactic biopsy if a lesion is visible on both mammography and US.

22   Which of the following is true regarding bone scintigraphy?
   a   It should be performed only in prostate cancer patients who are symptomatic.
   b   It is more sensitive than plain X-ray to detect prostate cancer metastases.
   c   Accurately differentiates a fracture from metastases.
   d   Sclerotic metastases appear as 'hot' on bone scintigraphy.
   e   The 'flare effect' in breast cancer patients indicates disease progression.

23 The following statements regarding croup are true.
   a   Commonly presents with stridor.
   b   Typically presents at six months to three years.
   c   Commonest organism is haemophilus influenza.
   d   Causes narrowing of the supraglottic airway.
   e   A lateral view is more useful than the AP film in differentiating from epiglottitis.

24 Which of the following are common causes of free air seen under the diaphragm on erect CXR?
   a   ERCP.
   b   Five days post laparoscopy.
   c   Perforated peptic ulcer.
   d   Colonoscopy.
   e   Perforated sigmoid diverticulum.

25 A 30-year-old man is being investigated for unexplained anaemia. After normal OGD and colonoscopy the decision is taken to investigate his small bowel. Which of the following tests should be considered as the next step?
   a   MR enteroclysis.
   b   Barium meal.
   c   Barium swallow.
   d   Barium follow through.
   e   Mesenteric angiography.

26 A 72-year-old woman presents with chronic PV bleeding. Which of the following investigations should be considered to investigate this further?
   a   Transvaginal ultrasound.
   b   CT of the abdomen and pelvis.
   c   MRI of the pelvis.
   d   Pelvic radiograph.
   e   Hysterosalpingogram.

27 A 70-year-old man with an elevated PSA is found to have prostate cancer on needle biopsy. He is otherwise asymptomatic. Which of the following staging investigations should he undergo?
   a   Skeletal survey.
   b   PET.
   c   MRI pelvis.
   d   CT pelvis.
   e   Transrectal ultrasound.

28 Which of the following features favour a diagnosis of rheumatoid arthritis over osteoarthritis on plain radiographs?
a   Osteophyte formation.
b   Subchondral sclerosis.
c   Subluxations at the metacarpophalangeal joints.
d   Involvement of the distal interphalangeal joints.
e   Atlanto-axial subluxation.

29 A 50-year-old man is diagnosed with ureteric colic on CT. However, on follow up KUB the calculus is found to be radiolucent. Which of the following could the calculus be composed of?
a   Calcium oxalate.
b   Calcium phosphate.
c   Uric acid.
d   Xanthine.
e   Magnesium ammonium phosphate.

30 A 48-year-old presents with lethargy and non-specific symptoms of feeling unwell. CXR shows bilateral hilar enlargement. Which of the following should be considered in the differential?
a   Sarcoidosis.
b   Pulmonary arterial hypertension.
c   Lymphoma.
d   Histoplasmosis.
e   Thymoma.

31 A premature neonate born at 30 weeks gestation is found to have bilateral diffuse ground glass appearance in the lungs with low lung volumes. Which of the following are possible differential diagnoses?
a   Transient tachypnoea of the newborn.
b   Meconium aspiration.
c   Neonatal infection.
d   Respiratory distress syndrome.
e   Congenital diaphragmatic hernia.

32 Which of the following modalities are indicated in the initial investigation of the acutely injured trauma patient?
a   FAST scan.
b   AXR.
c   MRI.
d   CT.
e   Angiography.

33 In paediatric imaging, which of the following injuries are suggestive of NAI?
   a   Interhemispheric subdural haemorrhage.
   b   Toddler's fracture.
   c   Posterior rib fracture.
   d   Metaphyseal corner fractures.
   e   Linear skull fracture.

34 The following statements are true regarding positron emission tomography (PET).
   a   The modality is radiation free.
   b   Has a better spatial resolution than CT.
   c   Provides anatomical information only.
   d   Images are acquired within seconds of ^{18}FDG tracer injection.
   e   Can be combined with CT scanning in the same session.

35 The following statements are true regarding ultrasound.
   a   The modality is radiation free.
   b   Has a better spatial resolution for liver imaging than MRI.
   c   Doppler imaging can demonstrate blood flow.
   d   Post-processing often takes longer than the image acquisition.
   e   Often combined with PET for fused images.

36 Regarding screening mammography which of the following view(s) of the breast are taken as standard?
   a   Antero-posterior.
   b   Cranio-caudal.
   c   Lateral decubitus.
   d   Mediolateral-oblique.
   e   Postero-anterior.

37 Which of the following statements is true with regards to Paget's disease of bone?
   a   It is more common in females.
   b   Typically occurs in teenagers.
   c   Demonstrates cortical and trabecular thickening on plain radiographs.
   d   Can cause congestive heart failure.
   e   Can demonstrate increased uptake on bone scintigraphy.

38 Radiological signs of hyperparathyroidism include:
   a   Trabecular resorption causing a 'salt and pepper' like appearance of the skull.
   b   Widening of the SI joints.
   c   Brown tumours in the pelvis.
   d   Generalised osteopenia.
   e   Bone resorption particularly affecting the radial aspect of the middle phalanges.

39   With regards to a CXR performed post pneumonectomy, which of the following statements are correct?
a   Progressive increase in the size of the air bubble is normal.
b   Two thirds of the hemithorax fills with fluid in 4–7 days.
c   Mediastinal shift occurs towards the operated side.
d   Elevation of the hemidiaphragm is seen on the affected side.
e   Successive radiographs demonstrate filling in of the hemithorax.

40   A 13-year-old child falls from her bicycle and presents with elbow pain. Which of the following ossification centres should have formed by this stage?
a   Radial head.
b   Trochlea.
c   Olecranon.
d   Lateral (external) epicondyle.
e   Medial (internal) epicondyle.

41   Which of the following can cause a mismatched perfusion defect on a V/Q scintigram?
a   Pleural effusion.
b   Sarcoidosis.
c   Pulmonary embolism.
d   Polyarteritis nodosa.
e   Chronic bronchitis.

42   A 35-year-old man reports a sudden pain behind his right ankle whilst playing squash. A partial tear of his Achilles tendon is suspected. Which of the following modalities could be used to assess his tendon?
a   Ultrasound.
b   MRI.
c   Plain radiographs.
d   CT.
e   Bone scintigraphy.

43   A patient is undergoing investigation for hyperaldosteronism (Conn's syndrome). Which of the following investigations may be useful in differentiating a benign adrenal adenoma from a malignant lesion?
a   Ultrasound.
b   Abdominal radiograph.
c   MIBG scintigraphy.
d   MRI.
e   CT.

44 Which of the following are radiographic signs of a simple pneumothorax?
   a   Volume loss of the underlying lung.
   b   Visible pleural outline.
   c   Flattening of the diaphragm on the affected side.
   d   Deep sulcus sign.
   e   Mediastinal shift away from the affected side.

45 A patient presents with exercise induced left leg claudication. Which of the
   following modalities could be used to investigate this further?
   a   MR angiography.
   b   Ultrasound.
   c   Techentium labelled red cell study.
   d   CT angiography.
   e   Digital subtraction angiography.

46 A patient presents with facial numbness and headaches. An MRI of the brain is
   arranged, which shows an enhancing lesion lying entirely within the cavernous
   sinus. Which of the following nerves pass through the cavernous sinus?
   a   Oculomotor nerve.
   b   Trochlear nerve.
   c   Trigeminal nerve (2nd division).
   d   Trigeminal nerve (3rd division).
   e   Facial nerve.

47 Which of the following normal structures can demonstrate calcification on CT
   of the head?
   a   Pineal gland.
   b   Choroid plexus.
   c   Cerebellar vermis.
   d   Medulla oblongata.
   e   Habenular commissure.

48 A 50-year-old patient is admitted with shortness of breath. CXR shows marked
   opacification of the right hemithorax with mediastinal shift towards that side.
   Which of the following should be considered in the differential diagnosis?
   a   Pleural effusion.
   b   Consolidation.
   c   Central obstructing tumour.
   d   Previous pneumonectomy.
   e   Mesothelioma.

49 Which of the following tumours commonly metastasise to bone?
   a   Renal cell carcinoma.
   b   Prostate carcinoma.
   c   Hepatocellular carcinoma.
   d   Meningioma.
   e   Breast carcinoma.

50 Which of the following require the intravenous injection of a radioactive tracer?
    a   Bone scintigraphy.
    b   CT pulmonary angiogram.
    c   PET-CT scan.
    d   SPECT scan.
    e   V/Q scan.

ANSWERS

1 F, F, F, F, T

CT has superior spatial resolution. MRI sequences take much longer to acquire, and as such are also prone to motion artefact from peristalsis and respiration (respiratory gating or breath hold techniques may help overcome this). MR contra-indications include permanent pacemakers and (ferromagnetic) metal stents / coils / fixation devices, and cochlear implants, as well as claustrophobia. MRI does not involve ionising radiation and offers better soft tissue differentiation than CT.

2 T, F, F, T, T

US is non-invasive, does not involve ionising radiation and is the first line investigation for suspected cholecystitis, biliary colic or obstructive jaundice, and acute renal failure. It is also useful in the assessment of cirrhosis, pyelonephritis, UTI, suspected renal tumours, liver lesions / metastases, DVT, inguinal hernias, vascular assessment (e.g. AAA, carotid dopplers), and palpable superficial lumps. The US waves do not penetrate bone and travel poorly through air, thus assessment of lung parenychma, bowel (unless fluid-filled) and bone is limited.

3 F, F, T, F, F

Although a skeletal survey involves 20 standard views, the radiation dose is significantly lower than a bone scan. A bone scan involves injection of the tracer and a return for imaging four hours or more later. Bone scans are more sensitive and can detect fractures occult on plain film, but are less specific (infection, inflammation, some tumours, and growth plates will also show increased uptake). Multiple fractures of differing ages are suspicious for NAI: bone scans are poor at determining fracture age, whereas fractures undergo set plain film changes over time as healing occurs.

4 F, F, F, F, T

At 16 weeks, abdominal shielding should be able to prevent most radiation from reaching the foetus during CTPA examination, however, with V/Q scanning the 'perfusion' radionuclide is injected and circulates intravenously, which exposes the foetus to radiation. Typically a 'half-dose' perfusion only V/Q scan is used when such a study is performed which is a lower dose to the mother than CTPA. D-dimer levels are likely to be (non-specifically) raised in pregnancy and are unlikely to be of any value. Pulmonary angiography is invasive and is now rarely used in any setting. Bilateral Doppler US is a routine part of the work-up for suspected PE in many hospitals because no radiation is involved and the local pressure of the foetus is known to be a risk factor for causing IVC or bilateral iliac / femoral vein thrombosis (along with the 'hyper-coagulable' risk of pregnancy itself).

5 F, T, T, F, T

Investigations are useful if the results will affect clinical management (i.e. confirm or excluding a diagnosis), or if they aid risk stratification of a condition. According to recent RCR recommendations, the following suspected diagnoses are appropriate indications for requesting an abdominal X-ray:

- Acute abdominal pain warranting hospital admission and surgical consideration.

- Acute abdominal pain: if perforation or obstruction suspected.
- Acute small or large bowel obstruction.
- Inflammatory bowel disease of the colon: acute exacerbation.
- Palpable mass (indicated in specific circumstances).
- Constipation (indicated in specific circumstances).
- Acute and chronic pancreatitis.
- Suspected ureteric colic / stones (indicated in specific circumstances).
- Renal failure.
- Haematuria.
- Foreign body in pharynx / upper oesophagus (indicated in specific circumstances).
- Smooth and small foreign body, e.g. Coin (indicated in specific circumstances).
- Sharp / poisonous foreign body.
- Blunt or stab abdominal injury.

Appendicitis is a clinical diagnosis in which plain AXR plays no role, however, US and CT may prove useful in equivocal circumstances.

Further reading
- Royal College of Radiologists. *Making the Best Use of Clinical Radiology Services: Referral Guidelines*. 6th ed. London: Royal College of Radiologists; 2007.

6 F, F, T, T, T
Prematurity is associated with respiratory distress syndrome due to a lack of surfactant in the lungs, PDA, germinal centre haemorrhage, periventricular leucomalacia, and necrotising enterocolitis. Meconium is the first stool passed; aspiration occurs if the meconium is expelled into the amniotic fluid prior to birth, or during labour and is more common in post-mature births, in prolonged labour, and if there is foetal distress during labour. In addition, due to increased size of the baby, post-maturity is associated with birth trauma and its sequelae, e.g. developmental dysplasia of the hip.

7 F, T, F, T, T
Extradural haematomas usually result from trauma and 90% are arterial bleeds into the space between the skull and the dura. They are biconvex in shape as their expansion is stopped by the sutures, where the dura is tightly attached to the skull. The pterion region is relatively weak and overlies the middle meningeal artery, thus 70–80% of extradural haematomas occur in the region of the temporal bone. A subdural haematoma is typically crescentic and is highly suggestive of NAI in children due to shaking-type injury.

8 T, T, F, T, F
Crohn's disease can affect any part of the GI tract, and 'skip lesions' with intervening areas of normal bowel are a typical feature; UC is typically contiguous from the rectum. Strictures are far more commonly seen in Crohn's; toxic megacolon can be present in either condition, but is more commonly seen in UC. Crohn's disease is more commonly associated with the following extra-intestinal manifestations: peripheral, migratory, non-deforming seronegative arthropathy, iritis, gallstones

and erythema nodosum. UC is associated with sclerosing cholangitis and pyoderma gangrenosum.

9 T, F, F, F, T
Abnormal mucin in the gallbladder and malabsorption of bile acids in CF patients with pancreatic insufficiency leads to an increased incidence of gallstones. Due to air trapping, the lungs in CF are hyperexpanded, which can produce a pectus carinatum appearance (as in asthma). The sweat has high sodium and chloride levels, with a value > 60 mmol/L of chloride in the sweat being consistent with a diagnosis of CF (the basis of the 'sweat test'). Meconium ileus, not meconium plug syndrome, is associated with CF. Meconium ileus is the presenting feature in approximately 15% of CF patients (thick meconium causes bowel obstruction), but 80% of cases of meconium ileus occur in CF patients. Meconium plug syndrome is neonatal bowel obstruction due to colonic inertia which usually occurs in term babies born to diabetic mothers; there is no association with CF. Pneumothorax is common and may be recurrent, due to rupture of bullae / blebs.

10 F, T, F, T, T
The optimal investigation for bladder tumours is direct visualisation +/− biopsy at cystoscopy, ultrasound (if the patient can tolerate a full bladder) is better than CT from a radiology perspective. OGD is the best method of investigation for gastric cancer; CT is known to have a poor sensitivity for this diagnosis. CT is the best means of staging the majority of intra-abdominal cancers. It is good for demonstrating complications of pancreatitis and, although often the first line investigation for suspected pancreatic cancer, is not as good as endoscopic ultrasound (EUS) in this regard. If available, a low dose non-contrast enhanced CT is the preferred method of investigation for renal colic, and radiation dose is comparable to that of an IVU.

11 F, F, T, F, T
There may be overlap and differences in individual UK centres as to which group of clinicians perform which procedures. Cardiologists perform coronary angiography +/− angioplasty and echocardiograms (essentially 'ultrasound of the heart'). Gastroenterologists or upper GI surgeons are likely to perform an ERCP; radiologists perform percutaneous-transhepatic cholangiopancreatography (PTC), rarely radiologists may perform ERCP. Radiotherapy is usually performed by clinical oncologists with additional training in radiology. Aside from interpreting films, radiologists perform a number of interventional procedures. Examples include US or CT-guided biopsies and drain placements, (non-cardiac) angiography, vascular stent placement, vascular embolisation, nephrostomies and trans-renal ureteric stent placement.

12 T, F, T, F, F
Gallstones are found in 12% men and 24% women overall, but the prevalence increases with age (commonest = female, fair, fat, forties, fertile). Gallstones are the second commonest cause of pancreatitis in the UK (alcohol is first), and cause approximately one third of cases. Only 10–20% of those with gallstones become

symptomatic. Three types of stones are recognised: pure cholesterol stones (15%), mixed stones (80% – probably a variant of cholesterol stones), and pigment stones (5%). Approximately 90% of renal stones are radio-opaque, but only 10% of gallstones are radio-opaque.

13 T, F, F, F, F

Forward tilting the head helps to elevate the larynx and reduces the risk of aspiration. Thin fluids are more likely to be aspirated than thick fluids; pastes are safer. Gastrografin® has a high osmolality and can cause significant pulmonary oedema if aspirated. Mixtures of barium paste are usually used under controlled conditions. Lateral views are employed, contrast can be clearly seen passing anteriorly into the trachea on these views. Frontal views are unlikely to detect subtle aspiration, but contrast may be seen in the distal trachea or main bronchi. In patients with an unsafe swallow, gastrostomy tubes can be inserted as 'PEG' (percutaneous endoscopic gastrostomy) tubes – under endoscopic guidance, or 'RIG' (radiological inserted gastrostomy) tubes – radiologically inserted: the stomach is inflated via a nasogastric tube and, under fluoroscopic guidance, the gastrostomy is performed percutaneously. The former is still the more common method in most centres.

Further reading
- Gore RM, Levine MS, editors. *Textbook of Gastrointestinal Radiology*. 3rd ed. Philadelphia, PA: Saunders; 2007: 215–20.

14 F, F, F, T, F

Another cause includes a right diaphragmatic hernia, with liver causing the opacification. The other options are causes of increased density in a hemithorax with shift towards the affected side (others would include lymphangitis carcinomatosis and pulmonary agenesis / hypoplasia).

Further reading
- Chapman S, Nakielny R, editors. *Aids to Radiological Differential Diagnosis*. 4th ed. Philadelphia, PA: Saunders; 2003.

15 T, F, F, T, F

US can be used in early pregnancy (6–10 weeks) to confirm the presence and viability of the embryo, particularly following PV bleeding. The 11–14 weeks US is the 'dating scan' which is used to estimate the due date; this scan can also confirm the presence of twins and take measurements to screen for Down's syndrome. The 20–22 week scan is performed to check for anomalies and any evidence of intrauterine growth retardation. Amniocentesis and CVS are US-guided procedures than sample foetal cells to detect chromosomal abnormalities. CVS is performed at 10–13 weeks, around four weeks earlier than amniocentesis. The original estimated risk of amniocentesis-related miscarriage is quoted as 1 in 200, but these are out-dated and recent studies place the risk at around 1 in 600 (compared to the higher risk of 1 in 100 for CVS). The head circumference to abdominal circumference ratio has the highest positive predictive value for IUGR. The crown-rump length is used up to 12 weeks, after this time it is not accurate due to flexion of the embryo. The femur length or biparietal diameter is used from 14 weeks, they have similar degrees of accuracy, but are less accurate in the third trimester.

16 F, F, F, T, T
The interpretation of heart size and the pulmonary vessels depends on the patient's positioning and the way in which the image was acquired (projection). Chest X-rays are normally performed PA (posterior-anterior) in well patients. If an AP (anterior-posterior) film is taken, the film is placed behind the patient and, as the heart is located anteriorly, the beam has to travel further prior to exposure, producing a magnification effect. An adequate inspiration is indicated by being able to count six anterior ribs and 10 posterior ribs in the mid-clavicular ribs above the right hemidiaphragm. In a poor inspiration the heart appears larger and the vascular markings more prominent. In a supine film, the diaphragm is positioned higher and the same effects are seen. Portable chest X-rays are invariably performed AP and often the patient's condition means only a supine film is possible, thus it is very difficult to interpret cardiac size on such films. In emphysema the lungs are typically hyper-expanded, the diaphragms flattened and the heart elongated (appearing 'narrower'). Rotation will not affect the apparent heart size.

17 F, T, F, F, T
An avulsion fracture occurs when a tendon or ligament pulls off a piece of the bone. If the skin surface is broken the fracture is described as compound or open; if three or more fragments are present the fracture is described as comminuted. Delayed union describes fracture fragments failing to unite within the normal expected interval (age related and bone specific). Non-union describes failure of fracture union when the process of healing has completely stopped. Pseudoarthrosis describes a non-union in which a 'false joint' forms between the bone fragments; fibrous tissue covers the bone ends and a surrounding bursal sac forms.

18 F, F, F, T, T
Although plain film and CT involve radiation to the patient, once the study is complete, there is no radiation remaining. For nuclear medicine studies, radiopharmaceuticals are administered and the patient retains radiation whilst the tracer remains in the body; many radiopharmaceuticals are excreted into breast milk. The time for interruption, or even cessation, of breast feeding will depend on the amount of tracer administered and the half-life of the tracer. Breast feeding needs to be stopped for 24 hours after ^{99m}Tc-white blood cell scan and for one hour after an ^{18}FDG-PET scan. Breast-feeding is usually stopped for three weeks after administration of ^{131}I and ^{125}I, ^{22}Na, ^{67}Ga, and ^{201}T1 containing radiopharmaceuticals.

Further reading
www.insideradiology.com.au/pages/view.php?T_id=66&ref_info.

19 T, F, F, F, T
Meckel's diverticulum is a vestigial remnant of the omphalomesenteric (vitelline) duct. It is almost always on the anti-mesenteric border and is a true diverticulum, containing all three layers of bowel wall. Heterotopic tissue is present in 50%

(usually gastric) and is usually responsible for any symptoms. Diagnosis is difficult clinically and radiologically as features can be non-specific, however, nuclear medicine ^{99m}Tc-Pertechnetate studies are the most sensitive test (85%), the tracer is taken up by any ectopic gastric mucosa present within the Meckel's. The commonest presentation in symptomatic patients is with GI bleed (28%), followed by intussusception (13%), obstruction (11%), perforation (11%) and diverticulitis (6%). The 'rule of 2s' applies to Meckel's diverticulum:

- **2%** of the population.
- **2** years: most common age at presentation.
- **2×** more common in males.
- **2** feet from the ileocaecal valve (60–100 cm).
- **2** inches in length (3–5 cm).
- **2** tissue types common (gastric/pancreatic).
- **20%** of patients have complications.

Further reading
- Thurley PD, Halliday KE, Somers JM, *et al*. Radiological features of Meckel's diverticulum and its complications. *Clin Rad*. 2009; **64(2)**: 109–18.

20 F, T, T, F, T
Polyhydramnios is defined as > 1,500 cm^3 of amniotic fluid at term or a vertical depth of > 6 cm without encountering foetal parts / cord at US, incidence = 2%. Causes include: maternal diabetes, rhesus incompatibility, GI causes (oesophageal atresia or other high GI atresia), neural tube defects (anencephaly, encephalocoele), chest disorders (diaphragmatic hernias, pulmonary hypoplasia), twins, or idiopathic. Oligohydramnios is the presence of < 500 cm^3 of amniotic fluid at term, or a vertical depth of < 2 cm without encountering foetal parts / cord at US. Causes include premature rupture of membranes (most common), foetal death, bilateral renal anomalies (agenesis / dysgenesis / infantile polycystic kidney disease / posterior urethral valves / prune belly syndrome), and IUGR (reduced renal perfusion).

21 F, T, F, F, T
There is no evidence based data to support the use of ultrasound for screening. US is used to evaluate lesions palpate by clinical examination or non-palpable lesions detected at mammography. Anechoic lesions are cystic and are almost always benign. US can detect implant rupture (the 'ladder sign' can be seen), however, MRI is more sensitive and specific (the 'linguini sign' is seen). US-guided biopsy are preferential if possible, because the biopsy is performed 'real-time', additionally there is no radiation involved.

22 F, T, F, T, F
Bone scintigraphy is often used for pre-operative staging of asymptomatic patients with prostate cancer to look for occult metastases. It is more sensitive than plain films for detecting nearly all metastases, however, it lacks specificity: degenerative change, infection, fractures, metastases, and benign increases in metabolic activity (e.g. Paget's disease) will all cause 'hot spots'. Sclerotic metastases appear 'hot'; some

lytic metastases may not be detected by scintigraphy. The 'flare effect' refers to the apparent worsening of the bone scan picture after chemotherapy, due to healing bone in areas of metastases and is not due to disease progression (often bone scans will not be performed up to six months following chemotherapy for this reason).

23 T, T, F, F, T

Croup occurs at six months to three years, is viral in origin (RSV or parainfluenza virus), and narrows the sub-glottic airways, with oedema of the mucosa, resulting in partial airway obstruction. A rare form of 'membranous croup' is related to super-imposed bacterial infection, typically by S. aureus. Epiglottitis is a bacterial infection (Haemophilus influenzae), usually occurs in an older age-group than croup, and causes supraglottic narrowing, although in 25% there is additional subglottic narrowing which can mimic croup on frontal films. The oedematous narrowing of the subglottis can often be seen as a 'steeple' (or inverted 'V') sign on frontal neck films. A lateral neck film is useful for differentiating the two, as it can show thickened aryepiglottic folds associated with epiglottitis.

24 F, T, T, F, T

Perforation of a hollow viscus and post surgical changes are the two commonest causes of free intra-abdominal air. Uncomplicated ERCP may give rise to contained air within the biliary tree but not free air. Colonoscopy carries a small risk of bowel perforation, however in uncomplicated cases no free gas should be seen.

25 T, F, F, T, F

A barium follow through involves obtaining images after the patient has drunk barium containing contrast medium. Small bowel enemas, MR (and CT) enteroclysis are studies where images are obtained of the small bowel during instillation of contrast medium via a tube placed through the stomach and duodenum. Using this technique eliminates the effect of the pylorus in only allowing a small amount of contrast medium to pass at any given time, thereby meaning better quality images of subtle mucosal detail can be obtained when compared with a follow through. However these tests are necessarily more invasive in that a tube has to be passed via the nose into the distal duodenum. A barium swallow evaluates the pharynx, oesophagus and gastro-oesophageal junction. A barium meal evaluates the mucosa of the stomach. It has largely been superseded by OGD, and its role is usually restricted to cases where OGD is not possible. Mesenteric angiography is indicated in cases where there is active bleeding and negative endoscopy.

26 T, F, T, F, F

In post menopausal bleeding, ultrasound (often performed via a transvaginal route) and MRI are the initial investigations of choice. It can be difficult to accurately identify the structure of origin of a pelvic mass on CT. Plain radiographs are crude assessors of soft tissue masses. HSG is a fluoroscopic study using instillation of contrast medium to investigate the uterine cavity and fallopian tubes. It is most often performed in younger women with fertility problems.

27 F, F, T, F, F
MRI is the radiological investigation of choice for staging of local disease. CT and ultrasound are not as sensitive, although transrectal ultrasound is used to guide the needle biopsy for diagnosis. Bone scintigraphy is used to look for distant metastases. Prostate cancer has a particular tendency to spread to the bones, metastases are seen as foci of increased uptake on the scintigram. Classically, prostate metastases appear as sclerotic rather than lytic metastases on plain radiographs.

28 F, F, T, F, T
The characteristics of osteoarthritic change are osteophyte formation, loss of the articular cartilage leading to subchondral sclerosis and cyst formation, and loss of joint space. Subluxations particularly within the cervical spine and bones of the hand are more typical of rheumatoid arthritis. The DIP joints are characteristically spared in rheumatoid arthritis.

29 F, F, T, T, F
Between 70–80% of calculi contain calcium and are radio-opaque. Pure urate (5–10% of all calculi) and xanthine (rare) calculi are radiolucent as are calculi composed of matrix (rare calculi containing mucopolysaccharides or mucoproteins). Struvite (mixed stones) are typically associated with infection, particularly proteus and are usually radio-opaque.

30 T, T, T, T, F
Bilateral hilar enlargement is usually due to either lymphadenopathy or pulmonary artery enlargement. The causes of pulmonary arterial hypertension can broadly be divided into those related to intra-cardiac shunts, chronic pulmonary emboli, chronic lung disease and idiopathic pulmonary hypertension typically presenting in relatively young women. Causes of bilar lymphadenopathy include:

• Sarcoidosis.
• Lymphoma.
• Infective: particularly viral, primary TB (although rarely bilateral and symmetrical).
• Metastases.
• Histoplasmosis.
• Coccidiomycosis.
• Extrinsic allergic alveolitis.
• Silicosis.
• Chronic berylliosis.

31 F, F, T, T, F
RDS is a disease of premature infants which involves increased alveolar surface tension due to lack of surfactant from underdeveloped type 2 pneumocytes. The characteristic radiological findings are diffuse ground glass changes with low lung volumes. Treatment is with exogenous surfactant administered via an endotracheal tube. Neonatal infection can present in a similar way, typically due to β-haemolytic Streptococcal infection during delivery. In meconium aspiration the lungs may be of normal volume, or hyperinflated due to air trapping, additionally meconium

aspiration and TTN usually affect term babies. Congenital diaphragmatic herniae do not have the radiological findings described.

32 T, F, F, T, F
FAST (Focused assessment with sonography for trauma) examination refers to a rapid assessment of the abdomen with ultrasound in the emergency setting to look for free fluid. AXR and MRI have no role to play in trauma. CT is the radiological investigation of choice in thoracic and abdominal trauma. Angiography has a specific role to play in pelvic trauma with ongoing haemorrhage, it may be able to localise and treat an individual bleeding vessel.

33 T, F, T, T, F
The possibility of NAI should be considered when the history does not correlate with the injury, there is a delay in seeking medical attention or if there is a specific pattern to the injuries (e.g. cigarette burn). Fractures that are relatively specific for NAI in addition to those listed above include fractures of the sternum, scapula or spinous processes. Interhemispheric and posterior fossa subdural haematoma are associated with vigorous shaking of the infant. NAI is associated with branching, depressed or multiple skull fractures. A Toddler's fracture is a spiral fracture of the distal tibia which is relatively common in ambulatory toddlers.

34 F, F, F, F, T
PET uses radioactive tracer isotopes which decay by positron emission, the positrons annihilate when they meet an electron to produce high energy gamma rays which can be detected by the PET scanner. The tracer is taken up by the target, thus functional information is provided. Spatial resolution is poor, thus PET-CT scanners are now frequently used to provide additional anatomical information / localisation. ^{18}FDG is the most commonly used tracer and is taken up by many tumours, due to their increased glycolysis; the tracer is usually injected 45–60 minutes before image acquisition to allow clearance from the blood pool and hence reduce background 'noise'.

35 T, T, T, F, F
The spatial resolution of US is excellent for liver imaging, and is better than CT and MRI. Doppler imaging allows the demonstration of blood flow and is additionally useful for differentiating bile ducts (if dilated) from intrahepatic blood vessels, which both appear anechoic. Fused imaging is possible, particularly with MRI (another radiation free modality), but has not been used with PET or CT. Post-processing is rarely used in US, but is an essential element of PET imaging, for many MRI sequences, and to a lesser extent CT.

36 F, T, F, T, F
As with most forms of plain film imaging two views are required as standard. Screening mammography typically involves a view from above (the cranio-caudal or superior-inferior view) and an angled, oblique view (mediolateral-oblique), to include the tail of the breast. Supplemental views may be necessary in symptomatic or recalled patients, these include true lateral views, exaggerated cranio-caudal,

or compression and magnification views. Frontal (AP or PA) views will not be beneficial, as the entire chest will be included on the views; decubitus views are not routinely employed.

37 F, F, T, T, T
Paget's disease is a chronic progressive disease of osteoblasts and osteoclasts causing abnormal bone remodelling. It is uncommon before the age of 40. It has multiple phases: initially there is a lytic phase, where aggressive bone resorption occurs causing a 'flame like' appearance in long bones. This is followed by an inactive phase where new bone formation and sclerosis predominate; often, the two stages occur concurrently. It can be asymptomatic or sometimes presents with warm extremities. Serum alkaline phosphatase (but not serum calcium) levels are elevated. The pelvis is most commonly involved, other typical sites include the femora, the skull and the vertebrae.

38 T, T, T, T, T
Parathyroid hormone stimulates osteoclastic bone resorption. Hyperparathyroidism may be primary (due to adenoma or hyperplasia), secondary (in response to renal failure) or tertiary (autonomous production following secondary HPT). Clinically serum calcium levels are elevated. In addition to the features described, widening of the symphysis pubis and resorption of the distal end of the clavicle are also seen. Brown tumours are cyst-like lesions.

39 F, T, T, T, T
A progressive increase in the size of the air bubble, diaphragmatic flattening or mediastinal shift to the opposite side is indicative of a broncho-pleural fistula.

40 T, T, T, T, T
The acronym 'CRITOL' (Capitellum, Radial head, Internal (medial) epicondyle, Trochlea, Olecranon and Lateral (external) epicondyle) describes the order in which the ossification centres appear. The first usually appears at approximately six months, and all are expected to be present by the age of 11–12 years (earlier in girls than boys). The exact age at which these centres appear is not clinically important, however the order in which they appear is. In particular the fact that the trochlea ossification centre invariably forms after the internal epicondyle ossification centre is important. If the trochlea centre is seen but an internal epicondyle centre cannot be seen then an avulsion fracture of the internal epicondyle should be suspected.

Further reading
- Raby N, Berman LH, De Lacey G, editors. *Accident & Emergency Radiology*. 2nd ed. London: Elsevier, Saunders; 2005.

41 F, F, T, T, F
Pulmonary emboli cause perfusion defects that are not matched by ventilation defects, however it is important to remember that V/Q examinations should be interpreted in the appropriate clinical context. Other causes of perfusion mismatch

include vasculitides (such as polyarteritis nodosa), TB, fat or tumour embolus and post radiotherapy change. Ventilation defects with normal or less defective perfusion ('reverse-mismatch') can be caused by COPD, pneumonia, lung collapse of any cause or pleural effusion. Matched defects in both perfusion and ventilation can be caused by pulmonary infarct, chronic bronchitis, sarcoidosis and collagen vascular diseases.

42 T, T, F, F, F
A complete Achilles tendon rupture will often not require any imaging due to the characteristic history and examination findings. Partial tears are harder to diagnose and either ultrasound or MRI can be used. The approximate percentage of torn fibres is used to help decide on treatment in some centres.

43 F, F, T, T, T
Both CT and MRI can be used to characterise adrenal lesions. CT relies on either the lesion containing fat or the enhancement characteristics of the lesion: contrast washout of > 50% on 10 minute delayed imaging suggests an adenoma. MRI relies on a particular type of study called chemical shift imaging to characterise the lesion. MIBG scintigraphy is useful in the detection of neuroectodermal tumours such as phaeochromocytoma or neuroblastoma.

44 T, T, F, T, F
Small pneumothoraces can be difficult to spot on a frontal radiograph. A lateral decubitus view with the suspected side up, an expiratory film or CT may be helpful. The deep sulcus sign is seen on supine radiographs where the anterior costophrenic angle is sharply delineated. Mediastinal shift away from the affected side and flattening of the diaphragm on the affected side are signs of tension pneumothorax (not a simple pneumothorax), a life threatening emergency that requires immediate decompression.

45 T, T, F, T, T
With regards to investigation of the peripheral vascular system, a variety of options are available. DSA is the gold standard and has the advantage that therapeutic intervention can be performed at the same sitting, however the test is necessarily invasive and there is a risk of bleeding or arterial dissection. Duplex ultrasound is cheap and non-invasive and can be used to estimate the degree of stenosis, but it is operator dependent. CTA and MRA both use i.v. contrast medium (gadolinium for MRA) to highlight the vessels. CTA employs ionising radiation. MRA does not and also has the advantage that images can be acquired in any plane, however the images take longer to acquire than CTA. Nuclear medicine studies lack the spatial resolution needed to detect stenotic vessels, however they can be used to investigate occult bleeding in the abdomen.

46 T, T, T, F, F
The cavernous sinus contains the following cranial nerves: oculomotor nerve (CN III), trochlear (CN IV), the first and second divisions of the trigeminal nerve (CN V1 and CN V2), and the abducens nerve (CN VI).

Further reading

- Moore KL, Dalley AF, editors. *Clinically Oriented Anatomy*. 5th ed. Philadelphia, PA: Lippincott Williams and Wilkins; 2005: 914.

47 T, T, F, F, T

Other normal structures that can calcify include the falx cerebri and tentorium, the thalamus, the dentate nuclei and arachnoid granulations. Pathological causes of calcification include vascular causes such as atherosclerosis and aneurysms and tumours such as meningiomas and oligodendrogliomas.

48 F, F, T, T, T

A large pleural effusion will displace the mediastinum away from the midline, although smaller ones may leave the mediastinum centrally placed. Mesothelioma and consolidation should not affect the position of the mediastinum. A central obstructing tumour can cause collapse of the lung causing opacification with mediastinal shift towards the affected side. The appearances are similar to those seen post pneumonectomy.

49 T, T, F, F, T

Although many different tumour types can metastasise to bone, the commonest include lung and thyroid in addition to those mentioned. In women breast cancer is the commonest cause of sclerotic bone metastases (breast metastases may be lytic or mixed also); in men, prostate cancer is the commonest cause. Other primary tumours that produce sclerotic metastses include carcinoid, lymphoma, medulloblastoma, colorectal adenocarcinoma, bladder TCC, pancreatic cancer, and neuroblastoma (in children).

50 T, F, T, T, T

Nuclear medicine studies involve the injection of a radioactive isotope. This tracer is linked to a targeting molecule, and emits radiation which can be detected. Importantly, the patient 'remains radioactive' for a time after injection, this depends on the half life of the tracer and how quickly the tracer is excreted from the body. The patient can therefore expose close contacts to radiation, of particular concern to caring mothers, or if breast feeding, and ward patients may need to be isolated. The PET part of the PET-CT scan requires a tracer injection. Although CT and plain X-ray use radiation to acquire images, no tracer needs to be injected and the patient does not continue to emit radiation after the study has finished.

Chapter 6
Extended matching item (EMI)

QUESTIONS

1 Theme: upper limb trauma

A   Bankart type fracture
B   Barton's fracture
C   Bennett's fracture
D   Chauffeur's fracture
E   Colle's fracture
F   Galeazzi fracture
G   Hill-Sachs type fracture
H   Nightstick fracture
I   No fracture
J   Monteggia fracture
K   Smith's fracture

Match the type of injury shown to the above fracture type.

a   A 63-year-old woman falls onto her outstretched right hand. Wrist X-rays are performed.

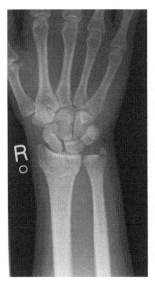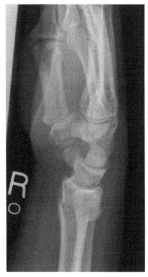

What type of fracture, if any is present?

b A 35-year-old man complains of right shoulder pain after falling. X-rays are taken.

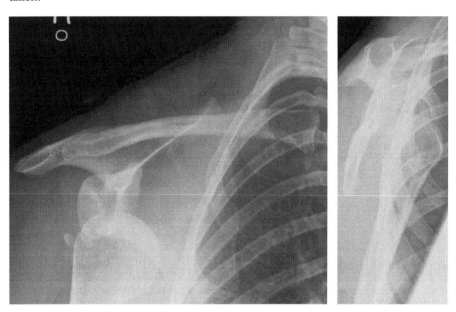

What type of fracture, if any is present?

c A 23-year-old man falls off his bike. On examination there is an obvious deformity of the forearm. An X-ray is performed.

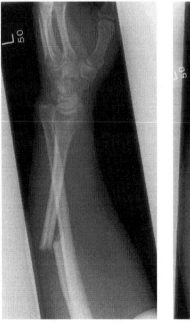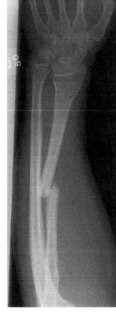

What fracture type is seen?

2 Theme: investigation of anaemia

A   Abdominal X-ray
B   Angiodysplasia
C   B12 levels
D   Barium enema
E   Barium follow-through
F   Barium meal
G   Barium swallow
H   Coeliac serology
I   Colonoscopy
J   Colorectal carcinoma
K   Erect Chest X-ray
L   Folate levels
M   Folate deficiency
N   Intrinsic factor levels
O   No imaging
P   Oesophago-gastric duodenoscopy
Q   Parietal cell antibody titres
R   Pernicious anaemia
S   Thalassaemia
T   Video capsule endoscopy

Choose the appropriate options from the list above to answer the following questions.

A 52-year-old man presents to his GP feeling tired, blood tests show Hb 11 g/dl, MCV 72 fL. The patient is referred for further investigation.

a   List two likely causes for this presentation.
b   Which blood test is it important to perform next?
c   List two first line imaging investigations.

Initial imaging investigations and further blood tests reveal no abnormalities. Following initial correction of the anaemia, the patient is followed up in clinic and blood tests are within the normal range.

d   What is the next most appropriate imaging step?

3 Theme: radiological signs

A   Boutonniere deformity
B   Celery stalk sign
C   Coffee bean sign
D   Double bubble sign
E   Finger in glove sign
F   Golden 'S' sign
G   Lead pipe sign
H   Rugger jersey spine
I   Stepladder sign
J   Swan-neck deformity sign
K   Terry Thomas sign
L   Z-shaped thumb

Match the descriptions below to the above listed radiological signs.

a   A sign associated with a deforming arthropathy, with DIPJ hyperflexion and PIPJ hyperextension.
b   A sign classically associated with a primary lung tumour which causes additional collapse of the adjacent upper lobe.
c   Sign found in an X-ray taken in neonates who present with bile-stained vomit, which is indicative of a diagnosis of duodenal stenosis.

4 Theme: what examination is being performed? Part 1

A   Abdominal X-ray
B   Barium follow-through
C   Bone scintigram
D   Computed tomography (CT) scan
E   Endoscopic retrograde cholangiopancreatography (ERCP)
F   MAG3 renal study
G   Magnetic resonace cholangiopancreatography (MRCP)
H   Percutaneous transhepatic cholangiogram
I   T1-weighted MRI
J   T2-weighted MRI
K   Ultrasound
L   Ventilation-perfusion (V/Q) scintigram

Match the options above to the investigations displayed.

a

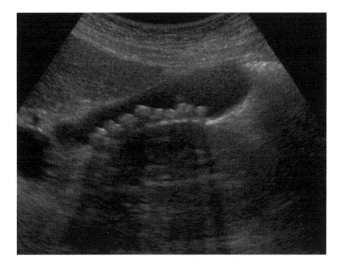

b

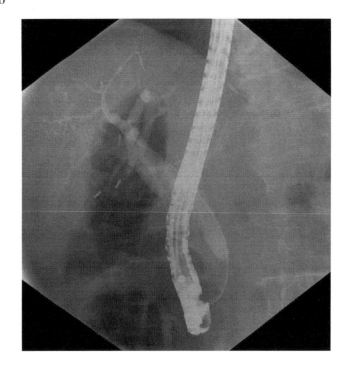

c

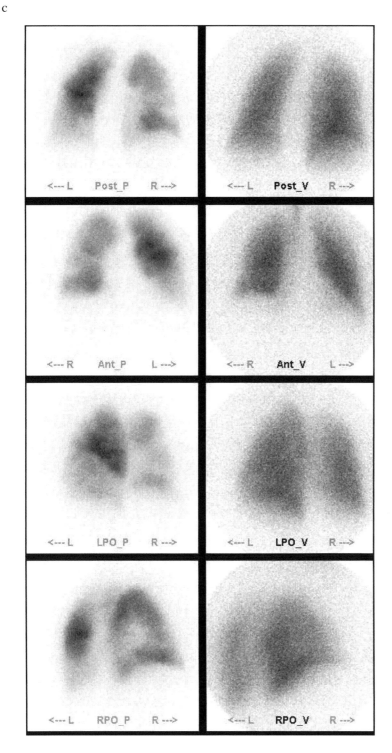

5 Theme: radiological findings in the phakomatoses

A   Ataxia telangiectasia
B   Gorlin syndrome
C   Incontinentia pigmenti
D   Neurofibromatosis type 1
E   Neurofibromatosis type 2
F   Sturge-Weber syndrome
G   Tuberous sclerosis
H   von Hippel-Lindau disease
I   Wyburn-Mason syndrome

Match the radiological findings listed to the relevant phakomatosis listed above.

a   CT abdomen shows cysts within the pancreas, multiple bilateral cystic and solid lesions within the kidney and bilateral irregular solid adrenal lesions. MRI head shows a cystic / enhancing lesion within the cerebellum.

b   MRI head shows a strongly enhancing extra-axial lesion in the fronto-parietal region and bilateral enhancing lesions within the vestibulocochlear nerves.

c   CT abdomen shows bilateral solid renal lesions which are seen to contain fat and enhance following contrast administration, and bilateral renal cysts. CT chest shows diffuse replacement of the lung parenchyma by thin-walled cysts measuring 2–20 mm in diameter, with a lower zone predominance.

6 Theme: inflammatory bowel disease

A   Barium enema
B   Barium meal
C   Barium swallow
D   Colorectal carcinoma
E   Distal interphalangeal joints
F   Ecthyma
G   Erythema nodosum
H   Fistulae
I   Flexible sigmoidoscopy
J   Impetigo
K   Knee joints
L   Magnetic resonance enteroclysis
M   Mesenteric angiography
N   Metacarpal joints
O   Primary sclerosing cholangitis
P   Proximal interphalangeal joints
Q   Pyoderma gangrenosum
R   Sacroiliac joints
S   String sign of Kantor
T   Toxic megacolon

A 17-year-old girl known to have Crohn's disease presents with increased bowel frequency, PR bleeding and abdominal pain. She is noted to have tender raised nodules on both shins. Initial abdominal X-ray is unremarkable.

a   What is the likely diagnosis of the noted skin lesions?
b   What is the most appropriate imaging investigation?
c   List two associations which are more likely to be present in Crohn's disease rather than ulcerative colitis?

A 37-year-old man with known ulcerative colitis presents with an acute exacerbation, with fresh blood passed PR.

d   What is the best first line imaging method?
e   List a complication of UC which can be detected by plain film
f   List two joints commonly affected with inflammatory bowel associated seronegative arthropathy.

7 Theme: what examination is being performed? Part 2

A   Abdominal X-ray
B   Barium enema
C   Barium follow-through
D   Barium meal
E   Barium swallow
F   Computed tomography (CT) scan
G   Intravenous urogram (IVU)
H   Kidneys-ureter-bladder (KUB) X-ray
I   Percutaneous transhepatic cholangiogram (PTC)
J   T1-weighted MRI
K   T2-weighted MRI
L   Ultrasound

Match the options above to the investigations displayed.

a

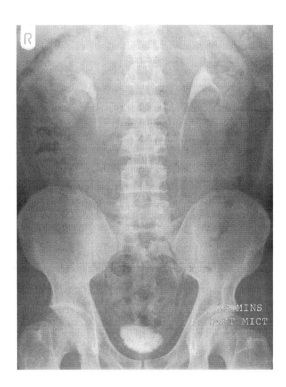

b

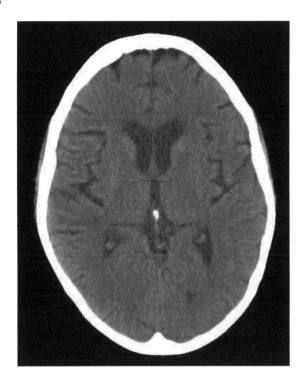

c

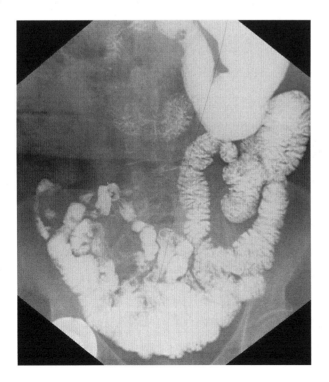

8 Theme: investigation of abdominal pain

A Angiography
B Appendicitis
C AXR
D Barium enema
E Barium follow-through
F Cholecystitis
G Coeliac disease
H CT
I CXR
J ERCP
K Gastroenteritis
L Intussusception
M Malrotation
N Meckel's diverticulum
O MRI
P No imaging
Q Pancreatitis
R Porphyria
S Renal colic
T Salpingitis
U Ultrasound

A 46-year-old woman with no past medical history, minimal alcohol intake and a non-smoker presents with acute epigastric pain. FBC, U&Es, LFTs, calcium and cholesterol are normal, amylase is 850 U/L. An abdominal X-ray and erect CXR are normal.

a   What is the diagnosis?
b   What is the most appropriate next investigation?

A six-month-old boy presents with vomiting and abdominal distension. History reveals that he has recently passed red jelly-like stool. The patient is haemodynamically well and the pain appears to settle in the department. AXR is normal.

c   What is the diagnosis?
d   What is the most appropriate next investigation?

A 27-year-old man is taken to A&E following a left abdominal stab wound. Initial observations: pulse 110, BP 98/58. He responds well to fluid resuscitation and is haemodynamically stable.

e   What is the optimal imaging investigation?

9 Theme: chest pathology

A   Anterior mediastinum
B   Left atrial enlargement
C   Left ventricular hypertrophy
D   Lingular lobe
E   Middle lobe
F   Middle mediastinum
G   Pericardial effusion
H   Posterior mediastinum
I   Right atrial enlargement
J   Right lower lobe
K   Right main bronchus
L   Right upper lobe
M   Right ventricular hypertrophy

Match the scenarios listed to the above options.

a   A man presents with shortness of breath. A CXR is performed, there are signs of pulmonary oedema, there is a double density at the right heart border, and the carinal angle is splayed to > 90°. What is the pathology described?

b   A 37-year-old man with known neurofibromatosis type 1 has a CXR performed for emigration purpose. The CXR shows a 3 cm mass forming obtuse angles medially with loss of the right paratracheal stripe, and splaying of the ribs. The hilar structures and right heart border are clearly seen through the mass. Where is the mass most likely to be located?

c   A 56-year-old women has had a recent course of antibiotics for a chest infection, but has not recovered. The GP requests a CXR, which shows an indistinct right heart border. The right hemidiaphragm is 3 cm higher than the left. A lateral film has not been taken. What structure has collapsed?

10 Theme: normal anatomical variants at CXR

A   Azygous fissure
B   Bifid rib
C   Bilateral cervical ribs
D   Fused ribs
E   Hemivertebrae
F   Inferior accessory fissure
G   Normal
H   Pectus cavinarum
I   Pectus excavatum
J   Pseudo-dextrocardia
K   Rib agenesis
L   Superior accessory fissure
M   Unfused epiphysis
N   Variant origin of the right subclavian vein
O   Wormian bone

Match the options above to the chest X-rays presented below.

a

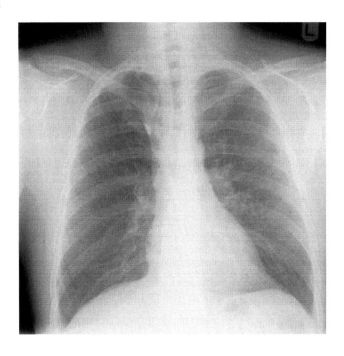

b

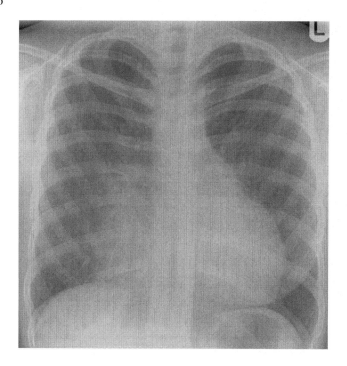

c

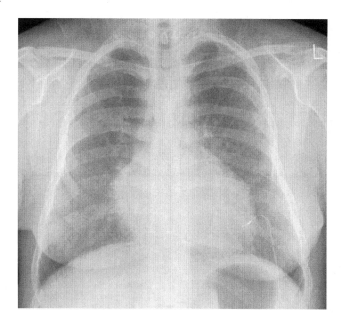

d

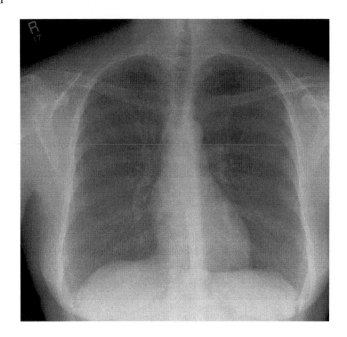

11 Theme: haematuria

A   24-hour urine for protein
B   Blood pressure
C   Contrast-enhanced CT (split dose)
D   Digital rectal examination
E   Intravenous urogram
F   Flexible cystoscopy
G   KUB X-ray
H   MRI
I   Non-contrast CT
J   Peak flow
K   PSA level
L   Serum creatinine
M   Ultrasound
N   Urine cytology
O   Urine dipstick

Match the clinical scenarios / questions below to the above list options.

a   A 48-year-old woman presents to her GP with macroscopic haematuria. She is normally fit and well, with no past medical problems. List two initial simple and relevant tests that can be performed by the GP.
b   A 42-year-old man presents with right loin-to-groin sharp pain which is intermittent. Urine dipstick shows red cells ++ and nil else, FBC is normal, serum creatinine is 280 µmol/L. What is the best imaging investigation to confirm the diagnosis?
c   Which test is key in establishing a diagnosis of nephrotic syndrome?
d   A 28-year-old man presents to the clinic with a single episode of painless haematuria, there is no history of trauma. Initial blood and urine tests are unremarkable. What two imaging methods would be most appropriate?

12 Theme: phaeochromocytomas

A   24-hour urine catecholamines
B   24-hour urine metanephrines
C   Adrenal medulla
D   CT adrenals
E   Dynamic contrast enhanced MRI
F   Extra-adrenal
G   Familial phaeochromocytosis
H ^{123}I-MIBG
I   MR spectroscopy
J   Multiple endocrine neoplasia type 1
K   Multiple endocrine neoplasia type 2
L   Neurofibromatosis type 1
M   Neurofibromatosis type 2
N   Plasma catecholamines
O   Plasma metanephrines
P   von Hippel-Lindau
Q ^{99m}Tc-MDP
R   Ultrasound
S   Zona fasciculata
T   Zona reticularis

Match the clinical scenarios / questions below to the above list options:

a   What is the commonest location of phaechromocytomas?
b   A patient has bilateral phaeochromocytomas, proven medullary thyroid carcinoma, and parathyroid adenomas. What is the unifying diagnosis?
c   A patient with VHL syndrome and a prior history of treated phaeochromocytoma is to be screened annually for phaeochromocytomas. What is the best method of doing this?
d   A phaeochromocytoma has been confirmed biochemically, but neither CT nor MRI demonstrates a tumour. What is the next best imaging investigation?

13 Theme: CT head examination

A   Cerebral contusion
B   Coup haematoma
C   Contra-coup haematoma
D   Diffuse axonal injury
E   Extra dural haematoma
F   Intraparenchymal haemorrhage
G   Intraventricular haemorrhage
H   Meningioma
I   Meningitis
J   Scalp haematoma
K   Subarachnoid haemorrhage
L   Subdural haematoma

Match the clinical scenario and imaging findings listed below to the above options.

a   A 56-year-old chronic alcoholic is admitted with reduced consciousness and possible fall. An unenhanced CT head is performed.

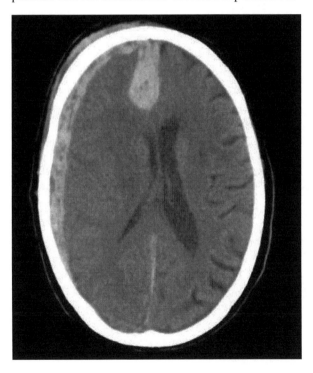

b   A 59-year-old man presents with severe headache, vomiting and reduced consciousness. A non-contrast enhanced CT head is performed.

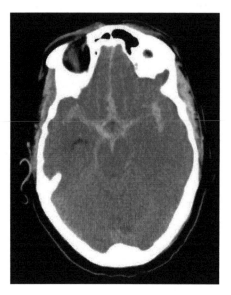

c   A 33-year-old man was admitted for severe H1N1-infective ARDS. He required treatment with extracorporal membrane oxygenation (ECMO) to maintain oxygenation. At day seven of treatment he is noted to have bilateral fixed dilated pupils. An unenhanced CT head examination is performed.

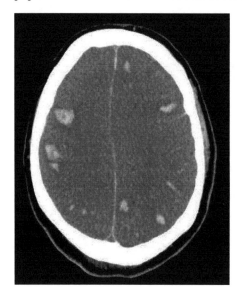

d   A 20-year-old man presents to A&E unconscious following a head injury
     sustained at an RTA.

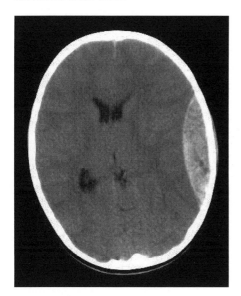

14 Theme: arthritides

A   Anti-double stranded DNA antibody
B   Anti-nuclear antibody
C   Bouchard's nodes
D   Boutonniere's deformity
E   Calcinosis
F   Jaccoud's disease
G   Felty's syndrome
H   Heberden's nodes
I   Hitchhiker's thumb
J   HLA-B27
K   HLA-DR3
L   HLA-DR4
M   HLA-DQ2
N   Opera glass deformity
O   Perinuclear anti-neutrophil cytoplasmic antibody
P   Reiter's disease
Q   Rheumatoid nodules
R   Sclerodactyly
S   Still's disease
T   Swan-neck deformity
U   Tophi
V   Ulna deviation

Match the clinical scenarios / questions below to the above list options.

a   A patient with known osteoarthritis complains of hard, painful swellings over a number of distal interphalangeal joints. Subsequent X-rays confirm bony outgrowths in these regions. What is the eponymous name of this finding?
b   A young patient suspected of having rheumatoid arthritis is found on examination to have a salmon-pink rash on her upper left arm, hepatosplenomegaly and lymphadenopathy. What is the likely unifying diagnosis?
c   A 25-year-old man presents with lower back pain and episodes of shortness of breath. A CXR shows mild biapical fibrosis, an X-ray of the lumboscaral spine shows bilateral sacroiliitis, with fusion of the lower lumbar vertebrae. Which major histocompatibility complex is most likely to be associated?
d   A patient presents systemically unwell. History reveals difficulty in swallowing and a history of Raynaud's phenomenon. On examination there is telangiectasisa around her mouth. An auto-antibody screen is positive for anti-centromere antibodies only. Hand X-rays are requested; list the two features that are most likely to be present.

15 Theme: lower limb trauma

A   Chest X-ray
B   Compartment syndrome
C   CT
D   Deep venous thrombosis
E   Fat embolism
F   Femur
G   Fibula
H   Foot
I   Maisonneuve
J   MRI
K   Osteomyelitis
L   Pilon
M   Posterior malleolus
N   Rhabdomyolysis
O   Ruptured Baker's cyst
P   Tibia
Q   Tillaux
R   Triplane
S   Ultrasound
T   Weber A
U   Weber B
V   Weber C
W   X-ray

Match the clinical scenarios / questions below to the above list options.

a   A 27-year-old male suffers a mid tibial fracture following a sports injury. The
     fracture is manually reduced and good alignment is seen. Four hours later he
     complains of increasing pain. On examination there is tense swelling of the calf,
     pallor of the foot and non-detectable dorsalis pedis and posterior tibial pulses.
     What is the likely diagnosis?
b   A 34-year-old man presents with knee pain following a sports injury. On
     examination there is a joint effusion and the anterior drawer test is positive.
     What is the best imaging investigation?
c   A 43-year-old woman slips, resulting in an external rotation injury to the ankle.
     On examination there is swelling medially. Ankle X-rays show a displaced
     transverse fracture of the medial malleolus of the distal tibia. Which additional
     X-ray should be considered?
d   Following a sports injury a patient complains of ankle pain. X-rays show a
     minimally displaced oblique fracture of the distal fibula, which extends inferio-
     medially to the level of the syndesmosis. What type of fracture is present?

16 Theme: chest X-ray

A   Left lower lobe collapse
B   Left upper lobe collapse
C   Lingular lobe collapse
D   Normal
E   Normal variant with azygous fissure
F   Pectus cavinarum
G   Pectus excavatum
H   Right atrial enlargement
I   Right lower lobe collapse
J   Right middle lobe collapse
K   Right upper lobe collapse
L   Right ventricular hypertrophy

Match the options above to the chest X-rays presented below.

a

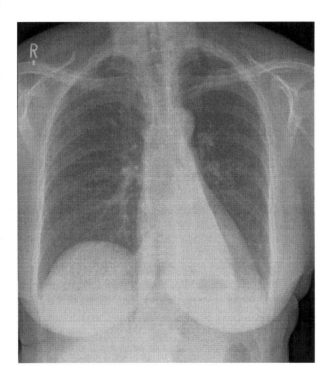

b

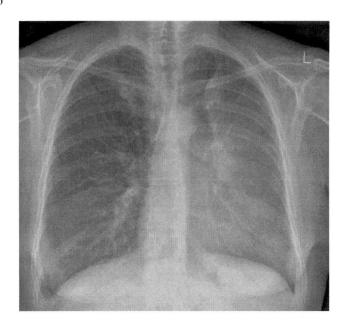

c

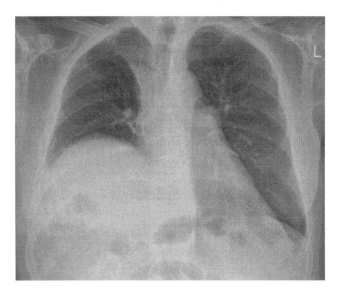

17 Theme: breast imaging

A Anterio-posterior
B Biopsy
C Chest X-ray
D Clinical examination
E Cranio-caudal
F Eggshell calcification
G FBC, U+Es, and LFTs
H Fine needle aspiration
I Galactography
J History taking
K Lateral
L Mammogram
M Medial-lateral oblique
N Microcalcification
O Milk of calcium
P MRI
Q Popcorn calcifcation
R Posterio-anterior
S Stereotactic mammography
T Ultrasound
U Wire localisation

Match the clinical scenarios / questions below to the above list options.

a A 32-year-old woman has had two close relatives diagnosed with breast cancer at a young age. Genetic screening shows her to be positive for the BRCA-1 gene. She needs to be screened annually for breast cancer, what is the most appropriate imaging method?

b A 36-year-old woman who has had breast implants inserted for cosmesis presents with pain over the right breast. The surgeon is concerned about rupture of the implant. What should you recommend for further assessment?

A 59-year-old presents to her GP with a recently detected lump in the left breast; she is referred to the rapid access breast clinic.

c What three elements comprise the triple assessment?

d If seen, which type of calcification pattern is the most suspicious for malignancy?

A 50-year-old asymptomatic patient presents for her first screening mammogram. There is no relevant family history.

e Which two views should be acquired as standard?

f A 3 cm mass is seen in the right upper outer quadrant, ultrasound confirms this to be solid. What is the best means of biopsying this lesion?

18 Theme: neonatal radiology

A   Barium enema
B   CT abdomen / pelvis
C   Cross-table lateral AXR
D   Erect CXR
E   Duodenal atresia
F   Hirschsprung's disease
G   Hyaline membrane disease
H   Inhaled foreign body
I   Left lateral decubitus AXR
J   Meconium aspiration
K   Meconium ileus
L   Meconium plug syndrome
M   Necrotising enterocolitis
N   Pyloric stenosis
O   Right lateral decubitus
P   Supine AXR
Q   Transient tachypnoea of the newborn
R   Ultrasound abdomen
S   Upper GI contrast fluoroscopy

Match the clinical scenarios / questions below to the above list options.

a   A six-hour-old baby born at 31 weeks is in respiratory distress with tachycardia, tachypnoea and cynaosis, and is using of the accessory muscles of respiration. CXR shows bilateral ground glass opacities with air bronchograms visualised and reduced lung volumes. What is the likely diagnosis?

A six-day-old ex-premature girl is noted to have an increasing abdominal distension. There are scanty bowel sounds on examination. An AXR shows dilated central loops of bowel, pneumatosis intestinalis, thickened bowel wall and portal venous gas.

b   What is the likely diagnosis?
c   The patient deteriorates further and the paediatric team are concerned about perforation, what X-ray view should you recommend to prove this?
d   A one-month-old boy presents with bilious vomiting and is in obvious distress. Bowel sounds are scanty. The paediatric surgical team suspect a diagnosis of malrotation. What is the best imaging study?

19 Theme: bone tumours

A 30-year-old man presents with knee pain following trivial trauma. An X-ray is performed and shows a pathological fracture within a 6 cm lesion in the distal femur. The lesion is predominantly lytic with a wide zone of transition. On the lateral view the periosteum is incomplete, with a raised periosteal reaction at both ends.

A   Askin tumour
B   Bone scintigram
C   Chest X-ray
D   Codman's triangle
E   CT abdomen and pelvis
F   CT knee
G   Ewing's sarcoma
H ^{18}FDG-PET
I   Lamellated
J   MRI knee
K   Osteoid osteoma
L   Osteosarcoma
M   Solid type
N   Sunburst

Match the clinical questions below to the above list options.

a   What is the most likely diagnosis given the imaging findings and the patient's age?
b   What is the type of periosteal reaction described?
c   What is the best initial investigation for assessment of the lesion?
d   List two most appropriate imaging examinations for staging.

20 Theme: abdominal X-ray

A Caecal bascule
B Caecal volvulus
C Duodenal atresia
D Gastric volvulus
E Giant diverticulum
F Large bowel obstruction
G Normal
H Sigmoid volvulus
I Sentinel loop
J Small bowel obstruction

Match the options above to the abdominal X-rays presented below.

a

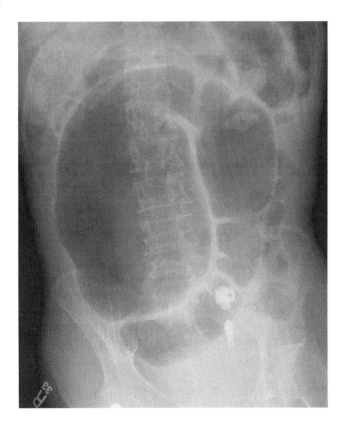

b

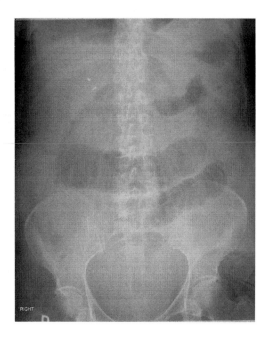

c

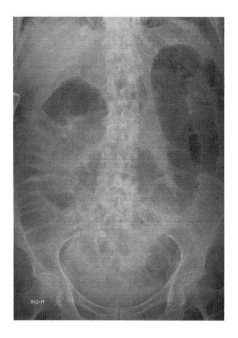

ANSWERS

1 Theme: upper limb trauma

a **B**

A fracture of the distal radius with associated dorsal displacement is termed a Colle's fracture ('dinner fork' deformity), but if this involves the joint line it is termed a Barton's fracture. In this case the joint line is clearly seen to be involved on the AP film, the lateral confirms the dorsal displacement. An addition minimally displaced fracture of the ulna styloid process is present, a common finding in Barton's or Colle's type fractures. A distal radius fracture with volar displacement is termed a Smith's fracture, if it additionally involves the joint line it is known as a Reverse-Barton's.

b **G**

There is an anterior dislocation of the shoulder joint – this is better appreciated on the 'Y' view, where the humeral head is seen anterior to the 'Y', overlying the thorax. See the below post reduction image to compare how a congruent gleno-humeral joint appears on the AP view. A Hill-Sachs lesion is a fracture of the upper outer aspect of the humeral head as it impacts the antero-inferior glenoid rim fracture following anterior dislocation of the shoulder. A tear of the labrum at the antero-inferior glenoid rim is termed a Bankart lesion.

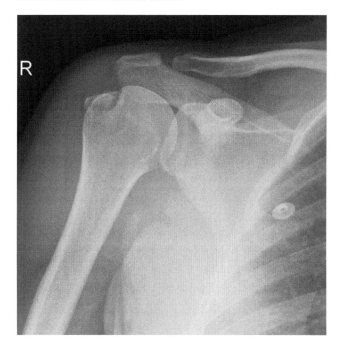

c **F**

A Galeazzi fracture is a fracture of the radius with associated dislocation of the distal radioulnar joint (*aide memoire* 'FROG': Fractured Radius Of Galeazzi); the radio-ulna dislocation is best appreciated on the AP film in this case. A Monteggia fracture is one of the proximal third of the ulna with associated dislocation of the head of the radius, *see* example below.

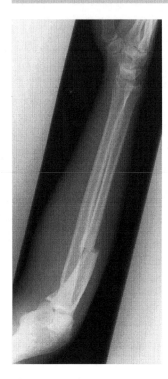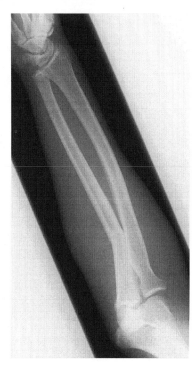

2 Theme: investigation of anaemia

a **B, J**, or **S**

The picture is of a microcytic, iron deficiency anaemia (IDA). IDA is confirmed by a low serum ferritin, red cell microcytosis or hypochromia in the absence of chronic disease or haemoglobinopathy. Normal range for MCV is 80-100 fL, normal Hb is > 12 g/dL (women), and > 13 g/dL (men). Causes include overt (GI, gynaecological, haemoptysis, etc.), or occult blood loss (GI, including NSAID use, oesophagitis, angiodysplasia), malabsoprtion of iron (coeliac disease, bowel resection), or haemoglobinopathies (sickle cell disease, thalassaemia). B12 or folate deficiency will cause a macrocytic anaemia.

b **H**

According to the BGS guidelines, all patients should be screened for coeliac disease, ideally by coeliac serology (anti-endomysial antibody or tissue transglutaminase antibody). Parietal cell antibodies are found in pernicious anaemia (associated with macrocytic anaemia due to lack of intrinsic factor and reduced B12 absorption).

c **P, D**, or **I**

Upper and lower GI investigations should be considered in all post-menopausal female and all male patients with IDA unless there is a history of significant overt non-GI blood loss. OGD is the preferred method of upper GI investigation and only the presence of gastric cancer or coeliac disease should deter lower GI investigation, which can be performed by colonoscopy or barium enema (BGS guidelines).

d O

Further direct visualisation of the small bowel is not recommended under BGS guidelines, provided the IDA is corrected and the Hb remains normal. If the patient remains transfusion dependent, small bowel investigation should be undertaken, enteroscopy may be helpful to detect and treat angiodysplasia. Video capsule endoscopy can be useful to look for angiodysplasia, small bowel radiological investigations are rarely useful unless there is a suspicion of Crohn's disease.

Further reading
* British Society of Gastroenterology *Guidelines for the management of iron deficiency anaemia*. British Society of Gastroenterology: www.bsg.org.uk/pdf_word_docs/ iron_def.pdf.

3 Theme: radiological signs

a J

The term 'swan-neck deformity' describes DIPJ hyperflexion and PIPJ hyperextension, Boutonniere deformity describes DIPJ hyperextension and PIPJ hyperflexion. It is classically described in theumatoid arthritis. There is only a solitary interphalangeal joint in the thumb.

b F

The Golden 'S' sign is named after Dr R Golden who first described the sign in 1925. It is classically described in relation to a central primary lung tumour, but may be seen with metastases or lymphadenopathy. There is right upper lobe collapse, with the lateral portion of the horizontal fissure concave inferiorly due to upward displacement and the medial portion convex inferiorly due to the mass, creating a (reversed) 'S' shape.

c D

The 'double bubble' sign describes the two 'bubbles' of gas seen in the upper abdomen on AXR located within the proximal duodenum and stomach. This is usually seen with duodenal atresia (which has an association with Down's syndrome). Rarer causes include annular pancreas, duodenal stenosis, a large choledochal cyst, Ladd's bands and a pre-duodenal vein. There is a lack of gas elsewhere in the bowel if the obstruction is absolute.

Regarding the other signs mentioned.

* Celery stalk sign – vertical striations extending longitudinally from the epiphysis through the metaphysis, usually seen in congenital rubella.
* Coffee bean sign – seen in sigmoid volvulus. The closed-loop sigmoid massively dilates, with the opposed bowel walls forming the apparent 'cleft' of the coffee bean.
* Finger in glove sign – sign of mucous plugging seen within bronchi. A non-specific finding, often found in cystic fibrosis and allergic bronchopulmonary aspergillosis.
* Lead pipe sign – loss of haustra resulting in a 'featureless' colon, often with associated narrowing of the colon, classically described in ulcerative colitis.

- Rugger jersey spine – described in osteosclerosis that is associated with the secondary hyperparathyroidism of chronic renal failure. Alternating bands of sclerosis and lucency are seen.
- Stepladder sign – an ultrasound sign of breast implant rupture, the equivalent findings on MRI are described as the 'linguini sign'.
- Terry Thomas sign – gap between the scaphoid and lunate bones (> 3 mm) seen on the AP view of the carpal bones, indicative of scapholunate ligament disruption.
- Z-shaped thumb – a deformity of the thumb classically seen in RhA, with hyperflexion of MCPJ and hyperextension at the IPJ. Also known as 'Hitchhiker's thumb'.

4 Theme: what examination is being performed? Part 1
a **K**
This is an ultrasound study of the gallbladder, which contains anechoic (black) bile fluid. There are multiple gallstones seen in this case, which cast an 'acoustic shadow', as the US waves do not pass readily through.

b **E**
The tip of the endoscope is seen within the duodenum, contrast is seen to pass retrogradely into the biliary system.

c **L**
This is a nuclear medicine V/Q lung scintigraphy study. The anatomy is not easily identified, but there are additional clues in the labelling: 'P' for perfusion, 'V' for ventilation. Multiple projections are acquired to aid diagnosis (posterior, anterior and left and right posterior-oblique views).

5 Theme: radiological findings in the phakomatoses
a **H**
VHL is a rare autosomal dominant condition associated with haemangioblastomas of the cerebellum, retina and spinal cord, renal cell carcinoma, phaechromocytomas, pancreatic cysts, and café-au-lait spots.

b **E**
The hallmark of NF-2 is bilateral acoustic neuromas (CNVIII lesions), which leads to deafness; cutaneous findings are uncommon. Other features include scoliosis, spinal cord schwannomas, and meningiomas (extra-axial). NF-1 features include Lisch nodules (hamartomas) of the iris, axillary freckling, cutaneous neurofibromas and café-au-lait patches. Radiological features include optic nerve gliomas, phaeochromocytomas, CNS hamartomas, peripheral nerve sheath neurofibromas, cortical thinning of the bones, scoliosis, dural ectasia, tibial pseudarthrosis.

c **G**
Peripheral features of TS include adenoma sebaceum, periungual fibromas, shagreen patches, and retinal hamartomas. CNS features include giant cell astrocytomas, cortical tubers, and sub-ependymal nodules. Other features include cardiac rhabdomyoma and

pulmonary cystic disease similar to lymphangiomyomatosis, renal angiomyolipomas (fat containing), renal cysts and, rarely, renal cell carcinoma and oncocytomas.

6 Theme: inflammatory bowel disease

a **G**

Eythema nodosum and pyoderma gangrenosum are associated with both Crohn's and UC. The described nodules are typical of erythema nodosum. The typical ulcerative form of pyoderma gangrenosum occurs in the legs, the atypical form is more superficial and occurs elsewhere on the body.

b **L**

MR enteroclysis is an excellent method for assessing complications of Crohn's, particularly in young patients where radiation exposure is more of a concern; X-ray screening is used to place an NJ tube for contrast instillation, but the dose is minimal compared to other studies). Barium follow through and small bowel enema studies are to an extent operator dependent and will not provide as good anatomical information, and have a relatively high radiation dose. CT enteroclysis can also be used, but the radiation dose means that the equivalent dynamic images acquired at MR are not feasible.

c **H, S**

There is an increased risk of colorectal carcinoma in both conditions, but there is a stronger association with UC. PSC is associated with UC; toxic megacolon is more common in UC. Fistulae, skip lesions and strictures (which can be seen as the 'string sign of Kantor' on Barium studies) are more common in Crohn's.

d **I**

UC starts distally and extends proximally. Generally in UC and particularly given the case presentation, direct imaging endoscopically is the best initial investigation.

e **T**

Abdominal X-ray can demonstrate signs of IBD such as mucosal oedema and thumb-printing, and complications such as obstruction or perforation; toxic megacolon is a complication of both conditions, but is more commonly seen in UC. Additionally, a featureless 'lead pipe' colon may be seen in UC.

f **K, R**

The commonest IBD-related pattern of arthropathy is that of an axial arthritis with sacroiliitis and spondylitis, followed by a large joint pauciarticular arthropathy (asymmetrical, typically involving the lower limbs).

7 Theme: what examination is being performed? Part 2

a **G**

The key finding is the presence of contrast media within the renal collecting systems, the ureters and bladder. An additional clue is given in the markers, this film was acquired 15 minutes post-micturition. A KUB film is a plain radiograph centred on the urinary system.

b **F**

The cranial bones are high attenuation on a CT study. In T2-weighted MRI the fluid within the ventricles will appear bright (high signal); in T1-weighting the fluid is of low signal intensity.

c **C**

The contrast medium is located centrally within loops of small bowel, making this a Barium follow-through. In an enema examination the contrast will be within large bowel, in a swallow study within the oesophagus and in a barium meal the stomach is distended with gas and coated with Barium.

8 Theme: investigation of abdominal pain

a **Q**

The markedly raised amylase is consistent with a diagnosis of pancreatitis. The WCC is normal and cholecystitis is less likely.

b **U**

There are numerous causes of pancreatitis, the commonest in the UK are gallstones and alcohol. US is the best investigation to look for gallstones and may confirm pancreatic inflammation. CT is useful to look for complications of pancreatitis further down the line, e.g. pancreatic necrosis, collections, or pseudocysts. Other causes of pancreatitis include steroids, hypercalcaemia, hypercholesterolaemia, mumps, autoimmune pancreatitis and post ERCP.

c **L**

Intussusception most commonly occurs from 3–12 months. 'Redcurrant jelly' stool is due to venous engorgement and ischemic mucosa leading to bleeding and mucous outpouring. Most cases are idiopathic in the younger age-group, and the majority are ileo-colic.

d **U**

Ultrasound has been shown to have a high sensitivity and specificity for detection. Reduction can be attempted by air enema or contrast enema under fluoroscopic guidance in the stable patient.

e **H**

The patient was initially unstable following a penetrating abdominal wound, but is now stable. There is a high suspicion of internal bleeding, CT is best to identify a source (renal, spleen, etc.). The unstable patient should have an emergency laparotomy. In certain circumstances angiography may be helpful to aid diagnosis or for treatment, following CT.

9 Theme: chest pathology

a **B**

The earliest sign is seen on a lateral view, or at barium swallow, with posterior displacement of the oesophagus. On a frontal CXR there is enlargement of the left atrial appendage, seen as an extra 'bulge' of the left heart border. There is also splaying / widening of the carinal angle (> 75°) and as the left atrium enlarges further it can be seen a 'double right heart border'. Isolated left atrial enlargement is most frequently seen in mitral stenosis, in which case, calcification may be seen in the region of the mitral valve.

b **H**

The obtuse angle formed with the mediastinum implies the mass originates within the mediastinum, loss of the paratracheal stripe is a further clue and the history is not of a patient at high risk for a primary lung tumour. The hilar structures are visible thus the mass is not located in the middle mediastinum (the 'hilar overlay' sign); the right heart border is visible which is against the mass being located in the anterior mediastinum. The splaying of the posterior ribs is further evidence of a posterior mediastinal location. The finding is an incidental one in an asymptomatic patient; the history of NF-1 suggests the lesion may well be a neurofibroma, which is in the differential of a posterior mediastinal mass.

c **E**

There is no left middle lobe, thus the right middle lobe is often referred to as simply the middle lobe. The middle lobe abuts the right heart border, thus complete collapse causes increased density / loss of this border. There is often associated loss of volume within the right hemithorax: the right hemidiaphragm is normally higher than the left, but ≤ 1.5 cm is the normal difference. The right middle lobe is more prone to atelectasis / collapse as its bronchus is narrow, has an acute angle take-off and is relatively long. Any lobar collapse may be secondary to infection, but in this age group, an obstructing tumour *must* be excluded, a follow-up CXR at six weeks should be arranged to ensure resolution, if there is any doubt, or a high clinical suspicion, a CT chest should be performed.

10 Theme: normal anatomical variants at CXR

a **A**

The presence of a normal variant, an azygous fissure / lobe, may cause confusion. This fissure appears in the region that the horizontal fissure is displaced to in RUL collapse (and the horizontal fissure is not always seen on a frontal radiograph).

b **I**

Pectus excavatum can mimic right middle lobe collapse, with the right heart border becoming indistinct, however, there is no associated volume loss, and if the patient is clinically well, RML collapse would be unlikely. The main clues are the horizontal orientation of the posterior ribs and the increased oblique angle of the anterior ribs (creating a number '7' shape on the left side). The lateral view (*see* below) can confirm the sternal depression, this may be marked and leave little room for the mediastinal structures (*see* CT image below).

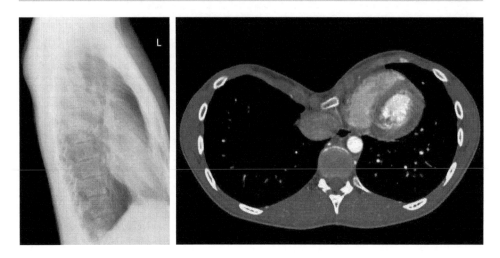

c **D**

There is fusion of the sixth and seventh right posterior ribs. This is usually an entirely incidental finding. Rarely fused ribs can cause dyspnoea due to their effect on respiratory dynamics, or scoliosis secondary to chest wall deformity. A bifid (bifurcated) rib is a single rib that splits into two, usually at the sternum. An example of a hemi-vertebrae is shown below, its presence may lead to scoliosis.

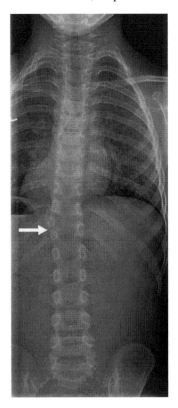

d **C**

Cervical ribs are congenital supernummery ribs arising from the seventh cervical vertebra. They are hypoplastic ('thinner') than normal ribs and can be seen as originating from the cervical vertebrae as these transverse processes are angled inferiorly (the transverse processes of thoracic vertebrae are angled upwards). Cervical ribs are associated with Klippel-Feil syndrome, overall the prevalence of a unilateral cervical rib is 0.2%, bilateral ribs are much rarer. They can result in morbidity by trapping structures between the cervical rib and scalenus muscle, examples include thoracic outlet syndrome, brachial plexus syndrome, or subclavian artery compression.

11 Theme: haematuria

a **B, O**

Urinalysis may confirm a UTI as a possible cause of haematuria. It is also useful to demonstrate the presence of protein if nephritis is a possibility. Blood pressure will be available in the GP surgery and is useful if chronic renal failure is suspected.

b **I**

The presentation is that of renal colic. KUB X-ray may show a calculus but lacks sensitivity and specificity and will not confirm the diagnosis. IVU has traditionally been used in diagnosis, however, this has been generally superseded by low-dose unenhanced CT abdomen/pelvis where available. In this case the high creatinine would make the use of contrast for an IVU more hazardous, thus unenhanced CT is unequivocally the better choice.

c **A**

Nephrotic syndrome is a defined by having proteinuria of > 3.5 g/day (per $1.73m^2$ of body surface area). There are numerous aetiologies.

d **F, M**

Macroscopic haematuria can be due to trauma, malignancy, stones, infection or glomerulonephritis. In patients < 30 years old with macroscopic haematuria the pick up rate of significant pathology is low (< 5%). Most will advocate ultrasound to assess the upper tracts as the first line investigation in this age group as it is radiation free. Flexible cystoscopy under local anaesthetic (or sometimes general) is the optimal method for assessing the lower tracts.

12 Theme: phaeochromocytomas

a **C**

Phaeochromocytomas arise from the adrenal medulla, originating in the chromaffin cells. The adrenal cortex consists of three zones: glomerulosa (aldosterone production), fasiculata (ACTH) and reticularis (cortisol). Approximately 10% of phaeochromocytomas are extra-adrenal (commonest = organ of Zuckerkandl), also 10% are bilateral, and 10% are malignant (which rises to 30% for extra-adrenal lesions).

b **K**

MEN-2a is associated with medullary thyroid cancer, phaeochromocytoma and parathyroid adenoma. MEN-2b is associated with the features of MEN-2a and a marfanoid phenotype. MEN-1 is associated with pancreatic tumours (insulinoma, gastrinoma, vipoma), pituitary adenomas, and parathyroid hyperplasia, but not phaeochromocytoma.

c **O**

Plasma metanephrine has a higher sensitivity (96%) but lower specificity (85%) compared to 24-hour urinary collection for catecholamines and metanephrines (sensitivity 87.5%, specificity of 99.7%). High-risk patients (those with a predisposing syndrome, or a family / personal history of a pheochromocytoma) are screened by the more sensitive plasma metanephrine testing. Patients at lower risk, but with suggestive symptoms (flushing spells, hypertension) are screened with the more specific 24-hour urine collection for catecholamines and metanephrines.

d **H**

^{123}I–MIBG is useful when phaeochromocytoma is suspected clinically and confirmed biochemically, but CT / MRI does not show a tumour. MIBG resembles noradrenaline and concentrates within adrenal or extra-adrenal phaeochromocytomas.

Further reading
*   Kudva YC, Sawka AM, Young WF Jr. The laboratory diagnosis of adrenal pheochromocytoma: the Mayo Clinic experience. *J Clin Endocrinol Metab*. 2003; **88(10)**: 4533–9.

13 Theme: CT head examination
a **L**

Acute haemorrhage appears hyperdense on non-contrast enhanced CT, as time continues the fluid attenuation matches that of the brain tissue, after seven days it becomes hypodense to brain parenchyma (the image below is from the same patient at six weeks). SDH is secondary to a tear of the bridging veins between the cortex and the draining venous sinus, resulting in haemorrhage into the inner meningeal layer of the dura. As they are venous bleeds, symptom onset may be slow. A crescent shaped hemorrhage forms, compressing the brain. It is medial to the skull, thus is not be bounded by the sutures, but they do not cross dural reflections (tentorium and falx) – as seen in this case, where the blood tracks to the right side of the falx, but does not cross to the left side. Elderly patients and alcoholic patients are particularly prone to this type of haemorrhage due to their increased cerebral atrophy.

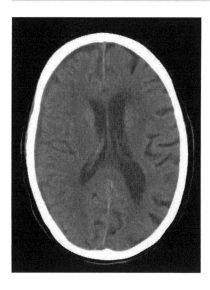

b **K**

SAH describes bleeding into the subarachnoid space (between the arachnoid membrane and the pia mater). This can occur spontaneously (typically following rupture of a cerebral aneurysm), or may be secondary to trauma. In this case haemorrhage (high attenuation in this non-contrast-enhanced CT) is seen within the circle of Willis. CT has a sensitivity of over 95% on the first day of SAH (lumbar puncture can confirm CT-occult cases), which reduces over time. In this case, a CT-angiogram study was performed, which can be reconstructed to demonstrate the aneurysm responsible for the bleed (*see* below). Direct DSA-angiogram can confirm this and also enable coiling of the aneurysm.

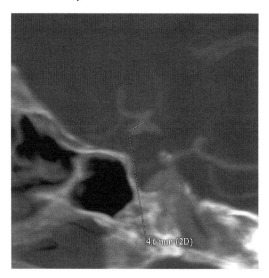

c **F**

ECMO provides cardiac and respiratory support oxygen in patients with severely damaged / diseased heart or lungs, often in the paediatric setting. Access is via large central vessels, and can be veno-venous or veno-arterial (e.g. the large bore cannulae in the right internal jugular vein in the below example in a patient with diffuse ARDS). Heparin is given for anticoagulation, this can result in intracranial bleeds as in this case. ECMO has been used for up to 10 weeks, survival on ECMO is around 60%, other complications include infection.

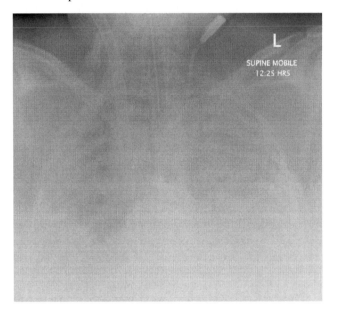

d **E**

EDHs are often caused by trauma and are usually arterial bleeds from the meningeal vessels between the dura mater and the cranium, resulting in a bi-convex haematoma; they do not cross the suture boundaries. The blood may accumulate rapidly due to the arterial origin, increasing intracranial pressure and causing compression, there is a 15–20% mortality, thus it is a neurosurgical emergency.

14 Theme: arthritides

a **H**

Heberden's nodes are seen in osteoarthritis, they begin as inflammation and pain at the DIP joints, which subsides to leave hard bony outgrowths; similar growths at the proximal interphalangeal (PIP) joints are termed Bouchard's nodes.

b **S**

Still's disease is characterised by rheumatoid arthritis, a salmon-pink rash, pyrexia, hepatosplenomegaly and lymphadenopathy; rheumatoid factor and anti-nuclear antibodies are usually negative. Felty's syndrome is defined by the presence of rheumatoid arthritis, splenomegaly, and neutropaenia; it affects < 1% of RhA patients.

c **J**

The features described are those of ankylosing spondylitis; 95% of these patients are HLA-B27 positive. Rheumatoid arthritis is associated with HLA-DR4. The three markers HLA-DR3, B8 and DQ2 are all associated with coeliac disease.

d **E, R**

CREST syndrome is a form of diffuse cutaneous scleroderma (systemic sclerosis); anti-centromere antibodies are associated and this form usually spares the lungs and kidneys. CREST comprises **C**alcinosis, **R**aynaud's disease, **E**sophageal dysmotility, **S**clerodactyly and **T**elangiectasia.

Further reading

- Balint GP, Balint PV. Felty's syndrome. *Best Pract Res Clin Rheumatol.* 2004; **18(5)**: 631–45.
- Bywaters EG. Still's disease in the adult. *Ann Rheum. Dis.* 1971; **30(2)**: 121–33.

15 Theme: lower limb trauma

a **B**

Compartment syndrome typically occurs following trauma, facture of the tibia is the commonest cause. Immediate surgery with fasciotomy is necessary to restore perfusion. The '5 Ps' of ischaemia are associated: pain, pallor, paraesthesia, paralysis, pulselessness. Venous pressure rises as intracompartmental pressure rises, when this rises above capillary perfusion pressure (> 30 mmHg) the vessels collapse and hypoxic injury occurs.

b **J**

The anterior drawer test is looking for stability in the anterior cruciate ligament. MRI is the best imaging investigation for assessment of ligamentous injury.

c **G**

The fibula and tibia essentially form a ring, thus an external rotation injury that results in a fracture of the distal tibia may also result in a fracture of the proximal fibula. The latter may be over-looked as the symptoms are centred on the ankle. Such a fracture combination is known as a 'Maisonneuve' fracture.

d **V**

The Weber classification relates to fibula fractures. Weber B fractures are those that are at the level of the tibia-fibular syndesmosis, Weber A fractures are below this and Weber C above (an isolated proximal fibula fracture is a subtype of this). Tillaux fracture is of the lateral tibial epiphysis in teenagers; pilon fractures are complex fracture of the distal tibia/fibula due to an axial load.

16 Theme: chest X-ray

a **A**

Left lower lobe collapse is often difficult to detect as it is 'hidden' behind the heart. There is compensatory hyperexpansion of the LUL, however, signs of volume loss are still likely to be present (raised left hemidiaphragm, inferior displacement of the left hilar structures and reduced volume of the left hemithorax). As in this case, a triangular shaped opacity can be seen behind the heart ('sail sign'), which can also give the appearance of a double left heart border. The left hemidiaphragm cannot be clearly seen medially, as collapse of the LLL onto this structure obliterates this 'silhouette sign'. Right lower lobe collapse has similar but opposite features, the 'sail sign' is often easier to appreciate as this is not 'hidden' by the heart (*see* below).

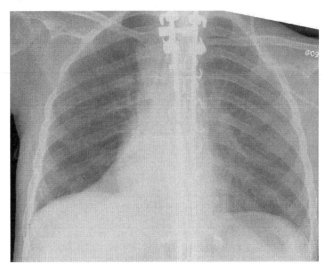

b **B**

Left upper lobe collapse appears as an increased hazy opacification ('veil-like') of the left upper zone. This appearance results due to compensatory hyperinflation of the LLL, thus there is aerated lung seen behind the collapse (*see* CT image below). There is usually significant volume loss with shift of the trachea to the left, reduced size of the left hemithorax and superior displacement of the left hilar point and hemidiaphragm. Additionally, as in this case, the apical segment of the LLL may herniated superiorly, giving a paradoxical clear outline to the aortic knuckle ('Luftsichel sign').

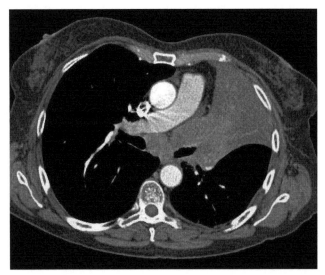

c **K**

Right upper lobe collapse; there is again volume loss. On the frontal film the horizontal fissure is seen to be displaced superiorly and medially. If the RUL collapse is secondary to a large obstructing tumour present, a reverse 'S' shape is seen, referred to as the 'Golden S' sign.

17 Theme: breast imaging

a **P**

Mammography has a radiation dose to be considered; furthermore it is less sensitive for diagnosing breast cancer in young patients with denser breasts. Ultrasound has not been approved for screening purposes. NICE recommends annual MRI screening for breast cancer in the following groups.

1   BRCA1 and BRCA2 mutation carriers aged 30–49 years.
2   TP53 mutation carriers aged 20 years or older.
3   Women aged 30–39 with an 8% 10-year risk of developing breast cancer and women aged 40–49 years with a 12% risk, i.e. those with the following family histories:
  •   Two close relatives diagnosed with average age under 30 years.
  •   Three close relatives diagnosed with average age under 40 years.
  •   Four close relatives diagnosed with average age under 50 years (providing all relatives are on the same family side and one is either the mother or a sister of the woman).

b **P**

Ruptures can present with pain, change in size/shape of the breast, leaking through the scar tissue, lymphadenopathy, or be silent. A study in USA reported the median implant age at rupture was 10.8 years; with submuscular implants being more likely to rupture than subglandular implants. It is advisable to remove ruptured implants; clinical examination is unreliable for detection, thus imaging is often essential pre-operatively. MRI if available is the most accurate imaging examination and can differentiate intracapsular (the 'linguini' sign) from extracapsular rupture; ultrasonography is a good alternative but its accuracy is operator dependent.

c **D, L** or **T, B** or **H**

Triple assessment comprises of clinical examination, radiological assessment (which can be by mammography or ultrasound or both, if relevant), and a pathological assessment (FNA for cytology, or biopsy for histology).

d **N**

There is an overlap in appearances of calcification, but microcalcification (areas < 1 mm), particularly in clusters is most worrying for malignancy. Linear, branching (intraductal) calcification is also suspicious. Popcorn calcification is coarse in nature and is associated with involuting fibroadenomas; eggshell (rim) calcification is typically seen in cysts or areas of fat necrosis; milk of calcium describes layering of calcium in microcysts. Dystrophic (irregular) calcification and calcification with a lucent centre are also more indicative of benign disease.

e **E, M**

These are the two standard screening views. Extra views may be required for completeness (true lateral, axillary tail, or extended cranio-caudal views), for better localisation ('rolled' views), or for additional information (magnified or compression views).

f **T**

If the lesion can be seen by ultrasound, this is the best method for biopsy, as it is 'real-time' and radiation free. Stereotactic mammography can be used if the lesion is occult by US, or just contains microcalcifications (e.g. DCIS). Both methods can be used to place wires to aid localisation for the surgeon if the lesion is not palpable clinically. MRI can be used for lesions occult at mammography and US.

Further reading

- NICE. *Familial breast cancer*. Guideline CG41: www.nice.org.uk/nicemedia/pdf/CG41fullguidance.pdf.
- Caskey CI, Berg WA, Hamper UM, *et al.* Imaging spectrum of extracapsular silicone: correlation of US, MR imaging, mammographic, and histopathologic findings. *Radiographics*. 1999; **19**: Spec No S39–51.
- Brown SL, Middleton MS, Berg WA, *et al.* Prevalence of rupture of silicone gel breast implants revealed on MR imaging in a population of women in Birmingham, Alabama. *AJR*. 2000; **175(4)**: 1057–64.

18 Theme: neonatal radiology

a **G**

Hyaline membrane disease is caused by pulmonary immaturity and insufficient surfactant production. The incidence decreases as babies approach term: present in 50% born at 26–28 weeks, and 25% at 30–31 weeks. The lungs are hypoinflated due to surfactant deficiency and hypoaeration (unless intubated), which helps distinguish it from the main differential diagnosis of meconium aspiration (more typically seen in post-mature babies), where the lungs are of normal volume or hyperinflated due to air trapping. The other findings are non-specific and may be present in both conditions.

b **M**

NEC is more common in preterm babies. Air in the bowel wall (pneumatosis intestinalis) is considered to be the AXR sign that is pathognomonic of NEC. Another feature is a 'fixed loop', a loop of bowel that does not move on serial radiographs. Treatment in the stable patient is conservative with bowel rest. Portal venous air does not have the same dire outcome as in the adult population, but free air requires surgical intervention.

c **I**

Left-side down decubitus is the optimal view, allowing detection of intraperitoneal air, which rises above the liver outline and can be seen more easily than on other views (right-side down is often more difficult due to air in the stomach or splenic flexure). An erect CXR is likely to be impractical in a neonate, particularly if unwell and / or ventilated.

d **S**

An upper GI contrast series is the study of choice in stable patients. A positive result is found if the duodeno-jejunal junction is not seen to cross the midline, to the left of the spine at a level higher than or equal to the pylorus, or if contrast ends abruptly or tapers in a corkscrew pattern. Lower GI series may show an abnormal placement of the caecum but this finding is less reliable.

19 Theme: bone tumours

a **L**

Osteosarcoma peak presentation is 20–30 years, the diaphysis of the femur is the commonest site affected, followed by the proximal tibia. Ewing's may have similar imaging features, but presents in a younger age-group: peak age is 15 years; 95% occur in those < 25 years. Askin tumours are part of the primitive neuroendocrine group of tumours and occur in the chest wall. Osteoid osteomas are benign tumours < 2 cm in size.

b **D**

Codman's triangle, lamellated ('onion skin'), and sunburst pattern are aggressive types of periosteal reaction. Codman's triangle occurs when a tumour grows too fast for the periosteum to respond with a complete covering of new bone, when seen laterally the raised ossification is seen forming an angle with the surface (not a complete triangle).

c **J**

The lesion is best assessed by MRI, which can give information on the soft tissue component of the tumour and the margins; ideally the MRI should cover the joints above and below the area involved in order to detect any skip lesions.

d **B, C**

Osteosarcoma typically metastasises to the lungs (lesions are ossified). CXR has been traditionally used; CT chest is now often used instead. Bone scans are useful for detecting skip lesions and metastases, the metastases will have the same characteristics as the primary tumour. Biopsies of suspected sarcomas should ideally be performed at a tertiary referral centre where the operation will take place, to avoid inadvertent seeding of the tumour.

20 Theme: abdominal X-ray

a **H**

The 'coffee bean' sign of sigmoid volvulus. There is a markedly distended loop of sigmoid colon, with distension resulting in loss of the haustral folds, which appears as an 'inverted U', with the apex pointing towards / overlying the RUQ. The bowel wall is oedematous, where these oppose each other centrally, a dense white line is formed – the groove of the coffee bean.

b **J**

The small bowel is predominantly located centrally. The valvulae conniventes are the mucosal folds of the small intestine and run circumferentially around the bowel. The upper limit of normal small bowel diameter is 3.5 cm. On an erect film there will be air-fluid levels seen, however, most AXR films are acquired supine, if there is significant fluid, the bowel dilation may not be easily discernable on such films. Causes of SBO include adhesional disease, hernias, intussusception and tumours. A sentinel loop is a focal area of small bowel thickening adjacent to an area of inflammation, e.g. near the pancreas in pancreatitis, or the RIF in appendicitis.

c **F**

The large bowel is located around the outer aspects of the abdomen. The mucosal folds of the large bowel are known as haustra. The maximal diameter of large bowel is 6 cm, although the caecum can expand up to 9 cm. Unlike with SBO, it is often easy to predict the level of obstruction from the plain film. In this case there is no gas within the rectum and there are clearly delineated dilated loops of sigmoid, descending, transverse and ascending colon; the transition point and level of obstruction lies within the distal sigmoid colon / rectum. The leading cause of LBO is a tumour; providing the ileo-caecal valve is competent there will not be associated SBO.

Chapter 7
Single best answer (SBA)

QUESTIONS

1   A 68-year-old woman presents with shortness of breath and pleuritic chest pain. She underwent an elective right total hip replacement 10 days previously which was uncomplicated. On examination the oxygen saturation is 88% (breathing room air) and there is a slight swelling of the right leg compared to the left. The D-dimer level is raised. What is the most appropriate first imaging investigation?
   a   Chest X-ray.
   b   CT-pulmonary angiogram.
   c   Pulmonary angiogram.
   d   Ultrasound bilateral lower leg veins.
   e   V/Q (ventilation / perfusion) scan.

2   A 48-year-old man is found to have a solitary pulmonary nodule on CXR. On CT, the 1cm lesion is rounded, well-defined and contains fat with central 'popcorn' calcification. What is the most likely diagnosis?
   a   Metastasis.
   b   Primary lung carcinoma.
   c   Pulmonary granuloma.
   d   AVM.
   e   Pulmonary hamartoma.

3   Which of the following results in the lowest radiation dose to an individual?
   a   A flight to Paris.
   b   Average UK background radiation for one year.
   c   Chest X-ray.
   d   Hand X-ray.
   e   Whole spine X-ray.

4   A 72-year-old smoker presents acutely with bilateral flank pain, which
    also radiates through to the back. He has a past medical history of angina,
    hypertension and diabetes. On examination there is a pulsatile central abdominal
    mass, BP is 110/60 and pulse is 95 bpm. What is the most appropriate imaging
    investigation?
    a   Abdominal MRI.
    b   Abdominal X-ray.
    c   Aortic angiogram.
    d   CT abdomen.
    e   Ultrasound.

5   A 56-year-old man has epigastric pain and reflux. The symptoms do not settle
    with anti-dyspeptic medication. Full blood count results show: Hb 9.3 g/dl,
    MCV 72 fl. What is the most appropriate investigation?
    a   Barium meal.
    b   Barium follow-through.
    c   Barium swallow.
    d   CT chest and abdomen.
    e   Oesophago-gastroduodenoscopy.

6   You suspect a patient of having suffered an intraperitoneal visceral perforation.
    Which of the following radiographic tests is the most sensitive for detection of
    free gas?
    a   Supine CXR.
    b   Erect CXR.
    c   Left lateral decubitus views.
    d   Erect AXR.
    e   Supine AXR.

7   A 43-year-old lady presents with right upper quadrant pain which radiates to the
    right shoulder. On examination the pain is reproducible on subcostal palpation
    and deep inspiration, but there are no other significant findings. Initial blood
    tests are normal. What is the most appropriate imaging test?
    a   AXR.
    b   Erect CXR.
    c   CT abdomen.
    d ^{99m}Tc-HIDA scan.
    e   Ultrasound.

8   A 46-year-old builder presents with abdominal pain, distension and vomiting. An abdominal X-ray is performed and confirms small bowel obstruction. A CT is requested; this demonstrates a loop of bowel which is seen to herniate medial to the inferior epigastric artery and lateral to the inguinal ligament. What type of hernia is present?
    a   Inguinal.
    b   Femoral.
    c   Richter's.
    d   Obturator.
    e   Spigelian.

9   A four-month-old girl has a proven first UTI. E. coli is cultured and there is a good response to antibiotics. What is the most appropriate way to proceed as regards imaging?
    a   Abdominal X-ray acutely.
    b   DMSA-scan within six weeks.
    c   MCUG within six weeks.
    d   No imaging.
    e   US within six weeks.

10 A 46-year-old woman presents with right upper quadrant pain. Blood results reveal an ALP of 460 IU/L and ALT of 90 IU/L. US shows multiple gallstones in a thin-walled gallbladder, prominence of the left hepatic bile ducts, an 8 mm diameter common duct and a 5 mm stone in the extrahepatic CBD. What is the most appropriate investigation to request?
    a   CT cholangiogram.
    b   Endoscopic cholangiopancreatogram.
    c   MR cholangiopancreatogram.
    d   Percutaneous transhepatic cholangiogram.
    e ^{99m}Tc-HIDA scan.

11 A 73-year-old patient is having difficulty with her swallow and is noted to have a 'choking' episode whilst eating on the ward. A fluoroscopic swallow is requested for further assessment. What would be the most appropriate contrast agent to use?
    a   Barium.
    b   Gastromiro®.
    c   Gastrografin®.
    d   Urografin®.
    e   Water.

12 Which of the following produces the highest radiation dose to an individual?
    a   Abdominal X-ray.
    b   A transatlantic flight.
    c   Average UK background radiation for one year.
    d   CT head.
    e   CT sinuses.

13 A 56-year-old man has an episode of expressive dysphasia which lasts a total of 30 minutes and has resolved by the time he presents to the A&E department. There is no relevant past medical history nor family history. Neurological examination is normal. What is the next appropriate management step?
   a   300 mg aspirin.
   b   Carotid Doppler imaging.
   c   Discharge with routine GP follow-up.
   d   Immediate CT.
   e   Immediate MRI.

14 A 62-year-old post-menopausal lady presents to the clinic with an episode of bleeding per vaginum. She is normally fit and well, and is not taking any medication. What is the most appropriate investigation?
   a   CT abdomen and pelvis.
   b   Dilatation and curettage.
   c   Hysterosalpingogram.
   d   MRI pelvis.
   e   Transvaginal ultrasound.

15 A 78-year-old woman has left hip pain following a fall. On examination the left hip is shortened and externally rotated. X-rays show a fracture of the left neck of femur. Which of the following fractures is at highest risk of avascular necrosis?
   a   Basi-cervical fracture.
   b   Inter-trochanteric fracture.
   c   Sub-capital fracture.
   d   Sub-trochanteric fracture.
   e   Trans-cervical fracture.

16 A 66-year-old woman presents with pain and stiffness within her hands; she has no systemic symptoms. She has minimal joint stiffness in the morning and the pain is aggravated by use, but relieved by rest. Hand X-rays reveal bilateral changes affecting the proximal and distal interphalangeal joints, with loss of joint space, subchondral cysts and sclerosis. What is the likely underlying diagnosis?
   a   Osteoarthritis.
   b   Calcium pyrophosphate arthropathy (pseudogout).
   c   Psoriatic arthritis.
   d   Reiter's syndrome.
   e   Rheumatoid arthritis.

17 An abdominal CT is performed in a patient with abnormal liver function tests. There is a solitary well circumscribed, homogeneous 4 cm lesion within the inferior aspect of the right lobe. The average Hounsfield unit value is 2. What is the most likely composition of this lesion?

a   Air.
b   Calcium.
c   Fat.
d   Fluid.
e   Soft tissue.

18 A five-year-old boy has had repeated episodes of sinusitis and has had three chest infections in the preceding six months. His GP sends him for a chest X-ray. The CXR shows no focal consolidation, but there is bilateral lower zone bronchiectasis; dextrocardia is also noted. What is the likeliest diagnosis?

a   α1-anti-trypsin deficiency.
b   Common variable immunodeficiency.
c   Cystic fibrosis.
d   Kartagener's syndrome.
e   Yellow nail syndrome.

19 A 28-year-old woman presents feeling generally lethargic, with joint pains, difficulty in breathing, and pain in both lower limbs. On examination she is found to have raised areas of erythema in both shins. Blood tests reveal an elevated serum angiotensin converting enzyme level. A CXR is performed and shows bilateral hilar lymphadenopathy but no focal lesions. What is the most likely diagnosis?

a   Churg-Strauss syndrome.
b   Histoplasmosis.
c   Non-Hodgkin's lymphoma.
d   Sarcoidosis.
e   Tuberculosis.

20 A 67-year-old man presents with left leg weakness with reduced sensation and milder, predominantly distal, left arm weakness. CT head shows low attenuation within the right medial frontal and parietal lobes. To which arterial territory does this correspond?

a   Anterior cerebral artery.
b   Middle cerebral artery.
c   Posterior cerebral artery.
d   Vertebral artery.
e   Superior cerebellar artery.

21 A 46-year-old man presents with dysphagia and weight loss. He is noted to have hyperkeratosis of the palms and soles. A barium swallow shows a tight, irregular stricture of the mid oesophagus. What is the most likely underlying diagnosis?
a   Psoriasis.
b   Epidermolysis bullosa.
c   Pemphigus vulgaris.
d   Tylosis.
e   Scleroderma.

22 A 13-year-old boy presents with a limp and associated right hip pain, there is no clear history of trauma. Only an AP film is performed and shows reduced height of the right femoral epiphysis, but normal alignment. The acetabulum is normal and the left hip is unremarkable. What is the most likely diagnosis?
a   Developmental dysplasia of the hip.
b   Perthe's disease.
c   Non accidental injury.
d   Slipped upper femoral epiphysis.
e   Transient synovitis.

23 Which of the following classifications of heart-to-viscera positioning has the lowest associated incidence of congenital heart defects?
a   Situs inversus / dextrocardia.
b   Situs solitus / dextrocardia.
c   Situs inversus / levocardia.
d   Situs solitus / levocardia.
e   Situs ambiguous.

24 A premature baby is born at 26 weeks gestation. Day 1 CXR shows widespread bilateral diffuse airspace opacification. Which of the following is the most likely diagnosis?
a   Congenital lobar emphysema.
b   Fallot's tetralogy.
c   Respiratory distress syndrome.
d   Congenital cystic adenoid malformation.
e   Meconium aspiration.

25 A 47-year-old man is found to have a mildly raised creatinine on routine blood tests. His GP refers him for a US for further investigation, which reveals a 4 cm irregular, echogenic mass in the right kidney. What is the next appropriate test?
a   CT abdomen.
b   Intravenous urogram.
c   KUB X-ray.
d   MRI abdomen.
e   Renal angiogram.

26 A 21-year-old man has a history of congenital right kidney pelvi-uretric junction obstruction. He is seen by a urologist, who wants to determine the split function and overall relative excretory function of each kidney. Which of the following tests is most appropriate?

a Ultrasound.

b Contrast-enhanced CT.

c IVU.

d ^{99m}Tc-DMSA.

e ^{99m}Tc-MAG3.

27 A 47-year-old woman presents with acute abdominal pain. On examination, there are signs of peritonism, with guarding and rebound tenderness. The surgical team review the patient and request an erect CXR in the first instance to look for evidence of a bowel perforation. What is the minimal volume of free air that needs to be present to be detected by this modality?

a 1 ml.

b 100 ml.

c 250 ml.

d 500 ml.

e 1000 ml.

28 A 75-year-old nursing home resident presents with abdominal pain and distension. AXR shows a large 'inverted U' shaped loop of large bowel extending from the pelvis with its apex projected over the right upper quadrant. The small bowel is not dilated. What is the likeliest diagnosis?

a Adhesional obstruction.

b Hernial obstruction.

c Sigmoid volvulus.

d Caecal volvulus.

e Acute diverticulitis.

29 A 30-year-old man presents with right loin pain and microscopic haematuria. Which of the following investigations is the optimal first line investigation?

a Unenhanced CT.

b Ultrasound.

c KUB.

d MRI.

e IVU.

30 A 12-year-old boy presents with a four-hour history of a red, swollen and exquisitely tender right testicle which is lying in a high, horizontal position. Which of the following is the next most appropriate step?

a Doppler ultrasound of the testicle.

b Nuclear imaging with technetium pertechnetate.

c Surgical exploration.

d Admission for serial examination.

e Admission for antibiotics.

31 Which of the following is the most commonly requested examination in a general UK hospital?
  a Abdominal X-ray.
  b CT abdomen.
  c CT head.
  d US abdomen.
  e Chest X-ray.

32 A patient is found to have a round, well defined 2 cm lesion within the right kidney on ultrasound. On CT the lesion is found to contain fat. What is the most likely diagnosis?
  a Renal cell carcinoma.
  b Oncocytoma.
  c TCC of the kidney.
  d Angiomyolipoma.
  e Renal infarct.

33 A 72-year-old man presents with a gradual decline with increasing cognitive impairment, memory loss and urinary incontinence. On examination there is no focal neurology, the patient has a broad-based shuffling gait and a stooped posture. A CT head is performed and shows ventricular prominence out of proportion to the sulcal atrophy, but no focal lesions. Lumbar puncture is performed with an opening pressure of 170 mmH$_2$O (normal: 70–180 mmH$_2$O), a protein level of 0.3 g/L (0.15–0.6 g/L), lymphocytes of 4/mm^3 (< 5/mm^3), and no growth on cultures. What is the most likely diagnosis?
  a Alzheimer's disease.
  b Multi-infarct dementia.
  c Normal pressure hydrocephalus.
  d Pick's disease.
  e Tuberculous meningitis.

34 A hand X-ray is performed in a six-year-old girl who has short stature and developmental delay, to check bone age. The film is noted to show shortening of the fourth and the fifth metacarpals, but no other abnormality. What is the likely diagnosis?
  a Hyperthyroidism.
  b Hypothyroidism.
  c Hyperparathyroidism.
  d Hypoparathyroidism.
  e Pseudohypoparathyroidism.

35 A 46-year-old man, with long-standing bronchiectasis, presents with burning
    joint pain of the fingers and swelling of the right wrist. On examination
    there is noted to be bilateral digital clubbing. An X-ray is performed and
    shows periosteal proliferation of new bone in the distal radius and ulna. The
    appearances are otherwise normal. What is the most likely diagnosis?
    a   Caffey's disease.
    b   Hyperparathyroidism.
    c   Hypertrophic osteoarthropathy.
    d   Osteoarthritis.
    e   Rheumatoid arthritis.

36 A 77-year-old man presents with gradually increasing right hip and thigh pain.
    There is no past medical history of note, although recently he has had problems
    with his hearing. An X-ray of the pelvis shows minimal loss of hip joint space
    bilaterally, thickening of the iliopectineal lines, with thickening of the right
    femoral cortex and coarsening of the trabeculae. The calcium and phosphate
    levels are normal, the alkaline phosphatase is raised. What is the most likely
    diagnosis?
    a   Hyperparathyroidism.
    b   Osteoarthritis.
    c   Osteoblastoma.
    d   Paget's disease.
    e   Prostate cancer metastases.

37 A 30-year-old asymptomatic man undergoes a CXR as part of a work medical.
    The radiograph demonstrates loss of clarity of the right heart border. Which of
    the following is the likeliest cause?
    a   Right lower lobe consolidation.
    b   Right upper lobe consolidation.
    c   Poor radiographic technique.
    d   Pectus excavatum.
    e   Right bronchial carcinoma.

38 A 22-year-old man presents with back pain. Plain films demonstrate fusion of the
    SI joints bilaterally with vertebral body squaring and ligamentous ossification in
    between the vertebrae. What is the most likely diagnosis?
    a   Reiter's syndrome.
    b   Psoriatic arthropathy.
    c   Ankylosing spondylitis.
    d   Scleroderma.
    e   Dermatomoyositis.

39 Which of the following does not form part of the left heart border on a frontal chest radiograph?
 a Left atrium.
 b Left atrial appendage.
 c Left ventricle.
 d Left main pulmonary artery.
 e Aortic arch.

40 A patient presents with change in bowel habit. Colonoscopy is attempted but it proves technically impossible to navigate beyond the sigmoid colon. Which of the following investigations would be best to perform next?
 a Targeted colonic ultrasound.
 b MR enteroclysis.
 c Abdominal X-ray.
 d CT colonography.
 e Barium enema.

41 What is the most appropriate investigation for the investigation of chronic lumbar back pain with no clinical or serological indicators of infection or neoplasia?
 a Myelography.
 b CT.
 c Lumbar spine radiograph.
 d Bone scintigram.
 e MRI.

42 A 55-year-old man presents several weeks after a fall complaining of a 'painful arc' when abducting his shoulder. MRI shows high signal intensity on T2 weighted imaging within one of the tendons of the rotator cuff. Which tendon is the least likely to be injured?
 a Supraspinatus.
 b Infraspinatus.
 c Teres minor.
 d Subscapularis.
 e Pectoralis minor.

43 A 38-year-old man presents with elbow pain after a fall. AP and lateral radiographs demonstrate the presence of an 8 mm anterior fat pad and a posterior fat pad. No obvious fracture line can be identified. Which of the following is most likely?
 a Ulna fracture.
 b No fracture.
 c Olecranon fracture.
 d Radial head fracture.
 e Humeral shaft fracture.

44 A 15-month-old child is found to have bilateral bowing deformities of the long bones of the leg along with widening of the growth plates. There is additional cupping and fraying of the metaphyses. What is the most likely diagnosis?
   a   Achondroplasia.
   b   Developmental dysplasia of the hip.
   c   Scurvy.
   d   Rickets.
   e   Perthe's disease.

45 Which of the following studies carries the highest effective radiation dose?
   a   CT head.
   b   High resolution CT chest.
   c   PET-CT of the abdomen and pelvis.
   d   CT KUB.
   e   CT colonography.

46 A 13-year-old overweight boy presents with chronic right hip pain. An AP radiograph shows minimal widening of the growth plate on the right side. What investigation should be performed next?
   a   Cross table lateral radiograph of the right hip.
   b   Frog leg lateral view of both hips.
   c   CT of the right hip.
   d   MRI of the right hip.
   e   Ultrasound of the right hip.

47 A 34-year-old man is involved in a high speed road traffic accident. He is conscious and is haemodynamically stable following fluid resuscitation. He complains of pain in his abdomen. Which of the following is the most useful imaging investigation?
   a   Abdominal radiograph.
   b   Erect chest radiograph.
   c   Ultrasound abdomen.
   d   MRI abdomen.
   e   CT abdomen.

48 A one-year-old boy presents with intermittent colicky abdominal pain, passage of 'redcurrant' stools and a palpable mass on the right side of the abdomen. Which of the following investigations should be performed to confirm the diagnosis?
   a   Ultrasound.
   b   CT.
   c   MRI.
   d   Small bowel follow through.
   e   AXR.

49 A 10-year-old boy presents with pelvic pain, swelling, tenderness and fever. Radiographs show a moth-eaten pattern of bone destruction and an onion-skin type of periosteal reaction. MRI demonstrates a large associated soft tissue component. What is the most likely diagnosis?
a   Fibrous dysplasia.
b   Chondrosarcoma.
c   Ewing's sarcoma.
d   Eosinophilic granuloma.
e   Lymphoma.

50 An 84-year-old smoker presents to the emergency department with hip pain. Plain films show an eccentric, poorly defined lytic area involving the left pelvis and acetabulum. What is the most appropriate investigation?
a   MRI pelvis.
b   CT pelvis.
c   CXR.
d   Follow up pelvic radiograph in six weeks.
e   Skeletal survey.

ANSWERS

1 a

The patient is at high risk for a pulmonary embolus, and 10–14 days post surgery is a classic time for presentation. The CXR is unlikely to diagnose a PE, but it forms an important fork in the diagnostic flow chart. A normal CXR makes a V/Q scan the next appropriate investigation, but an abnormal CXR necessitates a CTPA. The right leg swelling may be post-operative, but it still important to diagnose a PE over a DVT as most clinicians recommend a longer treatment period for the former. Pulmonary angiography is now rarely used for the diagnosis of PE.

2 e

There is a wide differential diagnosis for a solitary pulmonary nodule. These include neoplasm (primary and secondary), infection (including fungal), vascular, inflammatory, congenital and trauma. The commonest benign lesion is a granuloma which may or may not be calcified. Fat in a solitary pulmonary nodule is highly suggestive of a pulmonary hamartoma, as is the presence of 'popcorn'-like calcification.

3 d

The approximate effective dose from each of the listed options is as follows: (a) 0.004 mSv; (b) 2.23 mSv; (c) 0.02 mSv; (d) 0.001 mSv; and (e) 1.5 mSv. *See* introductory chapters for more information.

4 d

The average size of the abdominal aorta is 1.2–1.9 cm in women and 1.4–2.1 cm in men; a size > 3.0 cm is classified as AAA. The risk of spontaneous rupture is increased in smokers, diabetic and hypertensive patients, and also increases as the diameter of the AAA increases (particularly at ≥5 cm). In the stable patient, CT is the modality of choice to diagnose a leaking AAA. Non-contrast CT can show high density blood products from an acute bleed, and the leak may be localised following i.v. contrast. US can be used to diagnose AAA or monitor size change, but, in the acute situation, will not diagnose a leak. MR angiography can be used, but is limited by the acquisition time, image quality (compared to CT) and access to the scanner in the emergency situation in many hospitals. Interventional angiography can be used as an alternative to surgery in the stable patient for treatment / stent placement.

Further reading

* e-Medicine. Abdominal aortic aneurysm, rupture: www. emedicine.medscape. com/article/416397-overview.

5 e

The patient has upper GI symptoms, is in the high risk age group (> 50 years) and is found to have a microcytic (iron-deficiency) anaemia; MCV normal range = 80–100 fl. OGD is now the first line investigation, allowing direct visualisation of the mucosa, and biopsies can be taken. A barium meal can show the stomach in double contrast and may detect mucosal lesions, but diagnostic biopsies cannot be taken, thus a subsequent OGD would be necessary. Ba swallow can assess the oesophagus; Ba follow-through is a way to assess the small bowel; CT has low sensitivity for the detection of gastric tumours.

Further reading
* Goddard AF, James MW, McIntyre AS, *et al. Guidelines for the management of iron deficiency anaemia.* British Society of Gastroenterologists; May 2005: www.bsg. org.uk/pdf_word_docs/iron_def.pdf.

6 b

The erect CXR can detect as little as 1 ml of free gas under a hemidiaphragm. A left lateral decubitus view can be a useful adjunct in order to demonstrate free air around the liver.

7 e

The patient has features suggestive of cholecystitis or biliary colic; ultrasound is the first line radiological investigation. Without signs of peritonism or perforation, an erect CXR is not indicated. There is no role for AXR in the workup of suspected cholecystitis. CT can be considered if complications are suspected (gallbladder abscess / perforation), or if US is negative and a differential diagnosis is being considered. A ^{99m}Tc-HIDA scan is a more specialised investigation looking at biliary drainage or for a bile leak.

Further reading
* Royal College of Radiologists. *Making the Best Use of Clinical Radiology Services: Referral Guidelines.* 6th ed. London: Royal College of Radiologists; 2007.

8 a

Direct inguinal hernias originate infero-medial to the inferior epigastric artery and protrude through a weak point in the abdominal wall fascia. Indirect inguinal hernias originate supero-laterally to this artery, protrude through the deep inguinal ring and usually present in infancy. Spigelian hernias go through the spigelian fascia, the aponeurotic layer between the rectus abdominis muscle and the linea semilunaris. Femoral hernias pass through the femoral canal and obdurator hernias pass through the obdurator foramen.

9 e

NICE guidelines suggest that infants < 6 months with a first-time UTI that responds to treatment, should have an US within six weeks of the UTI. Children six months to three years old require no imaging unless atypical organisms are the cause. In those with recurrent UTIs a six week US and six month DMSA scan should be arranged. In those < 6-months-old with an abnormal US, or atypical organisms, or recurrent UTIs, an MCUG is performed.

Further reading
* NICE. *Urinary tract infection in children.* Guideline CG54. August 2007: www. nice.org.uk/CG54.

10 b

There is an obstructive pattern, with ALP (normal 30–115 IU/L) disproportionately higher than ALT (5–60 IU/L). MRCP is noninvasive and images the ducts without distention by injected contrast. ERCP carries a small but significant risk of pancreatitis, sedation reactions, contrast reactions, and perforation. However, in the described case ERCP has the advantage of being able to provide therapeutic intervention: stone removal should improve the patient's symptoms, relieve the hepatic obstruction and, furthermore, most surgeons prefer stone removal prior to planning an elective cholecystectomy. PTC is usually performed for therapeutic (stent placement, external drainage) rather than diagnostic purposes, when ERCP has failed or is unlikely to be successful; CT cholangiograms are rarely performed, and ^{99m}Tc-HIDA is used to assess biliary drainage.

Further reading
- Albert JG, Riemann JF. ERCP and MRCP – when and why. *Best Pract Res Clin Gastroenterol.* 2002; **16(3)**: 399–419.

11 b

Gastromiro® (iopamidol) is a water-soluble non-ionic contrast agent and is safest to use if aspiration is a risk. Gastrografin® (diatrizoic acid) is a high-osmolality iodine containing contrast agent, it is contraindicated if there is a risk of aspiration as, being hyperosmolar, it will cause prompt pulmonary oedema: likewise it should always be used with caution in paediatric patients as its presence in the bowel may lead to dehydration. Urografin® is a derivitive of gastrografin® without added flavouring (making it unpalatable). Barium aspiration can lead to a chemical pneumonitis; water will not be visible under fluoroscopy.

12 c

The approximate effective dose from each of the listed options is as follows: (a) 1 mSv; (b) 0.05 mSv; (c) 2.23 mSv; (d) 2 mSv; and (e) 0.6 mSv. *See* introductory chapters for more information.

13 a

The patient has had a transient ischaemic attack (TIA), some studies have shown that the risk of a stroke within four weeks is as high as 20%. The Rothwell classification counts a score of ≥ 4 counts as a high risk TIA, points are scored for each of:

- 1 point for age (≥ 60).
- 1 point for hypertension (≥ 140/90).
- 1 point for diabetes.
- 1 point for symptoms of 10–60 minutes and speech disturbance alone.
- 2 points for symptoms of > 60 minutes.
- 2 points for unilateral weakness.

The described patient scores 1 and is therefore low risk, but 300 mg aspirin should be started immediately in all cases, and measures for secondary prevention should be introduced. Recent NICE guidelines state that specialist assessment and investigation should be undertaken within 24 hours for high risk patients (seven days for low risk patients). MRI should only be performed if there is uncertainty over the diagnosis. Carotid Doppler imaging should be undertaken within seven days with a view to surgical endarterectomy (if appropriate) within two weeks.

Further reading

- Rothwell PM, Giles MF, Flossmann E, *et al.* A simple score (ABCD) to identify individuals at high early risk of stroke after transient ischaemic attack. *Lancet.* 2005; **366**: 29–36.
- NICE. *Stroke: diagnosis and initial management of acute stroke and transient ischaemic attack (TIA).* Guideline CG68. July 2008: www.nice.org.uk/nicemedia/ pdf/CG68NICEGuideline.pdf.

14 e

TV ultrasound is the first line investigation, looking for endometrial thickness and ovarian pathology. If the endometrium is thickening (most centres consider ≥ 5 mm as being abnormal in post-menopausal women) a D&C procedure will usually be the next step. MRI can be used to assess uterine or ovarian lesions; CT may be used for staging purposes. An HSG is usually performed for suspected uterine anomalies, or as a work-up for infertility.

15 c

Proximal femoral fractures are divided into subcapsular and extracapsular. The joint capsule runs from the acetabulum to the inter-trochanteric line anteriorly and to the junction of the middle / distal third of the femoral neck posteriorly. Thus intracapsular fractures are those of the femoral neck: sub-capital, trans-cervical and basi-cervical fractures, and extracapsular include inter-trochanteric, sub-trochanteric and femoral shaft fractures. Intracapsular fractures are more susceptible to AVN because the main supply to the femoral head is from the circumflex femoral arteries, which enter *via* the capsule and are more likely to be disrupted by such fractures. Additional blood supply from the ligamentum teres artery via the acetabular fossa and the retinacular branches on the surface of the femoral neck, are usually insufficient to prevent AVN. Furthermore they may be compromised by the raised pressure secondary to blood within the joint capsule post-fracture. The more proximal the subcapsular fracture, the greater the risk of vascular compromise, thus a sub-capital fracture has the greatest risk of AVN.

Further reading

- Schmidt AH, Swiontkowski MF. Femoral neck fractures. *Orthop Clin North Am.* 2002; **33**: 97–111.

16 a

Osteoarthritis can be primary (age-related) degenerative, or secondary (trauma, inflammatory conditions, osteonecrosis, haemochromatosis, calcium pyrophosphate disease). It typically affects the DIP and PIP and first CMC joints of the hand, the hips, knees, spine and first MTP joint, with sparing of the MCP joints, wrist, elbow, shoulder and ankles. Heberden's nodes are hard or bony swellings that affect the DIP joints; Bouchard's nodes are similar lesions affecting the PIP joints. Psoriatic arthritis can be a great mimic of any of the other forms of arthritis, but the lack of systemic symptoms is against this.

17 d

The Hounsfield unit scale (named after Sir Godfrey Hounsfield, the inventor of CT imaging) is a quantitative way of measuring the radiodensity of a material. Pure water is nominally given the value 0 and pure air the value –1000. These were chosen to allow a universal and easily available means of calibration. However, inherent noise means that even pure water will not have exactly 0 HU when scanned. The denser the material, the better it will attenuate ('block') the X-ray beam. Fat attenuates the beam less than water, soft tissue and bone attenuate it more, thus the respective values are fat –120, water 0, muscle 40, bone > 400. The composition of organs such as the liver changes with pathology (e.g. fat infiltration) and following the administration of contrast medium (increases as the contrast is dense). Most tissues of interest within the abdomen have similar Hounsfield values, thus narrow windows have to be used to accentuate this difference.

18 d

Congenital ciliary disorders are classified as primary ciliary dyskinesias (PCD). They have an autosomal recessive inheritance, with the primary cause being a dysfunction in genes encoding for dynein in the ciliary arm. When accompanied by the combination of situs inversus (approximately 50% of PCD), chronic sinusitis and bronchiectasis, it is known as Kartagener's syndrome. The term 'immotile ciliary syndrome' is not used, as sperm in affected men may retain motility.

Further reading
- e-Medicine. Pulmonology: Kartagener syndrome: www.emedicine.medscape. com/article/299299-overview.

19 d

Löfgren syndrome is a form of acute sarcoidosis with the triad of bihilar lymphadenopathy, erythema nodosum, and arthritis. It is associated with a good prognosis, with the majority having complete resolution of disease within two years. Serum ACE levels are often found to be elevated in sarcoid. The other listed options are all causes of bihilar lymphadenopathy.

Further reading
- Moore SL, Teirstein AE. Musculoskeletal sarcoidosis: spectrum of appearances at MR imaging. *Radiographics*. 2003; **23(6)**: 1389–99.

20 a

The ACA supplies the medial surfaces of the frontal and parietal lobes, the anterior four fifths of the corpus callosum, the anterior diencephalon, the frontobasal cerebral cortex, and the deep structures. Ischaemic anterior circulation strokes (areas supplied by the right and left internal carotid arteries and their branches) account for 70% of all cases – 90% of these occur in the MCA braches; ACA strokes are rare.

Further reading

• Rubin M, Safdieh JE, editors. *Netter's Concise Neuroanatomy*. Philadelphia, PA: Saunders; 2007.

21 d

Tylosis is one of the 'palmoplantar keratoderma' group of disorders. It has an autosomal dominant inheritance and is characterised by hyperkeratosis (thickening) of the palmar and plantar surfaces and oral leukoplakia. There is a strong association with SCC of the oesophagus (affecting 95% of patients by 70 years of age). Psoriasis does not have a known association with oesophageal cancer. The other skin conditions mentioned do not typically have hyperkeratosis as a feature, and are rarely linked to oesophageal malignancy. Epidermolysis bullosa is often associated with SCC of the skin; there are rare case reports of oesophageal cancer. Pemphigus has a rare paraneoplastic form, typically associated with lymphoma. Scleroderma results in oesophageal dysmotility, which predisposes to reflux – a risk factor for oesophageal cancer.

22 d

SUFE typically presents at 10–15 years and is bilateral in 15–25%. Early signs include widened growth plate and, on the AP view, reduced height of epiphysis (which slips posteriorly); the 'frogleg' lateral is more accurate for showing a medial slip. Perthe's disease (avascular necrosis) presents at 5–10 years, features include widened joint space and subchondral fissure fracture; later features include fragmented epiphyses, subchondral cysts, increased density, and OA. In DDH, the acetabulum would also be expected to be abnormal (too shallow). Transient synovitis presents at 5–10 years and is the commonest cause of a non-traumatic limp in this age group. US typically shows a joint effusion without synovial thickening. NAI typically presents before three years of age.

23 d

Normal anatomy is situs solitus/levocardia, which has the lowest association with CHD (< 1%). Complete reversal of all organs is known as situs inversus (4% asscoiation with CHD), reversal of some of the organs is called situs ambiguous, or heterotaxy (up to 100% asscoiation with CHD). Reversal of the organs, but normally sited heart: situs inversus/levocardia has a 95% CHD association. Isolated reversal of the heart with normally-placed viscera is termed situs solitus / dextrocardia (CHD in 95%).

24 c

'Respiratory distress syndrome' is a condition of premature infants, due to lack of surfactant production from type II pneumocytes, which leads to increased alveolar surface tension, causing a classical bilateral granular appearance. Treatment is with administration of surfactant via an endotracheal tube. Complications include pulmonary interstitial emphysema and bronchopulmonary dysplasia.

25 a

In the first instance, CT acquired pre-contrast and arterial and delayed post-contrast is optimal for further characterisation. Renal angiograms are only useful in specific circumstances and MRI would not be used as a first line imaging modality. Plain film is unlikely to add any information and IVU will not add more information than a CT.

26 e

GFR can be estimated by plasma sampling, using analogues of inulin, ^{99m}Tc-DTPA, or ^{51}Cr-EDTA. Alternatively, gamma camera methods can be used, with or without blood sampling, to estimate function from the quantity of tracer extracted from the plasma and excreted via the kidneys. ^{99m}Tc-MAG3 can be used to derive this tubular extraction rate and additionally information on the differential function between each kidney's filtration activity is acquired. ^{99m}Tc-DMSA is a 'static' renal agent that is useful for detection of post-pyelonephritic scarring in children. An IVU is a crude method for showing differences in the excretion of both kidneys and certainly cannot offer accurate percentage split function, likewise delayed acquisition post-contrast CT. US cannot show renal function.

27 a

In suspected perforation, the most useful and sensitive plain film investigation is the erect CXR (if the patient can co-operate), studies have shown that as little as 1 ml of free intrapertitoneal air can be demonstrated on an erect CXR. A supine AXR can detect free air, but the signs are subtle, an AXR obtained with the left side down (left lateral decubitus) position is also useful: the air rises and is then seen anterior to the liver.

Further reading
- Miller RE, Nelson SW. The roentgenologic demonstration of tiny amounts of free intraperitoneal gas: experimental and clinical studies. *Am J Roentgenol Radium Ther Nucl Med.* 1971; **112**: 574–85.

28 c

These appearances are highly suggestive of sigmoid volvulus. This accounts for approximately three quarters of colonic volvulus cases. Patients with elongated, dilated colons are prone to the condition. A relatively high incidence is seen in 'institutionalised' patients, where the lack of mobility and the medications used are regarded as risk factors. Caecal volvulus typically has its apex projected to the left of midline or to the left side of the abdomen. Adhesions and herniae are the commonest causes of small bowel obstruction. Diverticulitis can cause obstruction if an inflammatory mass forms, however the radiological findings are not typical of those described.

29 a

CT is now the investigation of choice for patients with suspected renal colic. Usually an unenhanced examination is sufficient. In cases where there is some doubt as to whether a calcific density lies inside or outside a ureter, a second delayed phase after the administration of contrast medium to outline the ureter may be employed. Ultrasound is useful for assessment of hydronephrosis or for investigation of other causes of haematuria but is less sensitive than CT at detection of calculi particularly within the ureter. KUB still plays a role in the follow up of radio-opaque calculi. MRI is not indicated. The advent of CT has meant that the IVU is now employed far less frequently when CT is available; its role now is limited to specialised situations such as the investigation of post-operative complications.

30 c

Although Doppler ultrasound is occasionally performed to examine Doppler flow to the testicle, it should never be allowed to delay immediate exploration in cases where there is a high index of suspicion for testicular torsion. Technetium imaging has fallen from favour with the rapid rise of availability of ultrasound along with the fact that there is an associated radiation dose in an often young group of patients.

31 e

The chest X-ray remains the most commonly requested examination in current UK practice. Familiarity and expertise in its assessment therefore remains of paramount importance to all clinicians.

Further reading
- De Lacey G, Morley S, Berman LH, editors. *The Chest X-Ray: a survival guide*. London: Elsevier, Saunders; 2007.

32 d

Fat within a well defined renal lesion is virtually diagnostic of an angiomyolipoma.

33 c

Normal pressure hydrocephalus has a classic triad of dementia, a gait abnormality, and urinary incontinence. The main differential diagnosis is Parkinson's disease which may present with similar features, but rigidity and tremor are normally present. NPH is a chronic communicating hydrocephalus where CSF formation eventually equilibrates with absorption, thus the intracranial pressure (and opening pressure at LP) is raised to the upper limit of normal, but typically does not produce clinical features of raised ICP (headache, nausea, vomiting). Clinical symptoms result from distortion of the central portion of the corona radiata by the distended ventricles.

34 e

Pseudohypoparathyroidism is a condition associated with primary resistance to PTH. Patients are short, have a rounded face, obesity and developmental delay, hypocalcaemia, short fourth and fifth metacarpals / metatarsals, and soft tissue calcification. Patients have low calcium, high phosphate and inappropriately high PTH. Symptoms may also be secondary to hypocalcaemia: carpo-pedal spasm, tetany, muscle cramps and seizures. Pseudopseudohypoparathyroidism has similar clinical phenotype, but the calcium levels are normal.

35 c

HOA can be primary or secondary to pulmonary, pleural (fibroma, mesothelioma), cardiac (cyanotic heart disease with right-to-left shunt), and abdominal (Crohn's) disease. It is sometimes known as 'hypertrophic pulmonary osteoarthropathy' (HPOA) due to the strong association with lung disorders, including: bronchogenic carcinoma, TB lung abscess, bronchiectasis, and emphysema. The exact mechanism of HOA is not known, theories include an increase in peripheral blood supply (due to a release of vasodilators not metabolised by the lung), or the presence of chemical irritants which initiate a periosteal response.

36 d

The aetiology of Paget's disease is unknown, but it is thought to be due to a viral infection (paramyxovirus) which may be present for years before symptoms occur; the disease is rare before the age of 40. There are three stages: osteoclastic stage (increased bone resorption), osteoclastic-osteoblastic stage (compensatory increased bone formation leads to disorganised deposition of lamellar bone), and 'burnt-out' stage. Hypertrophy of the bone can lead to nerve entrapment: hearing loss can occur if Paget's affects the skull bones around the inner ear. Sarcomatous degeneration and pathological fractures can occur in affected bones. Treatment is with bisphosphonates.

37 d

Loss of clarity of the right heart border implies a loss of the normal interface between air and soft tissue that would normally exist (the so-called 'silhouette' sign). Although this can represent right middle lobe pathology, in this instance, in a young asymptomatic patient, pectus excavatum should be considered.

38 c

Characteristically this affects young men. HLA-B27 is positive in 95%. The classic 'bamboo' spine appearance may be paired with arthritis of proximal joints such as the hips. AS is associated with inflammatory bowel disease, aortitis, and upper lobe pulmonary fibrosis.

39 a

The left atrium is the most posterior of the heart chambers and thus forms the posterior heart border on a lateral chest radiograph. The right heart border is formed by the right atrium.

40 d

CT colonography is a relatively new technique which involves bowel preparation and air insufflation via the rectum whilst a CT examination is performed. It has a good specificity and sensitivity for detection of colonic lesions (particularly those beyond 1cm in size) and is rapidly being employed across the country. Ultrasound is poor for colonic examination due to air casting an acoustic shadow. MR enteroclysis is an investigation of the small bowel. AXR has no role to play. Barium enema was the traditional investigation of choice for colonic lesions until colonoscopy became favoured, and still has a part to play, especially if CT colonography is not available.

41 e

MRI is now the preferred imaging modality for most spinal disease. Other modalities are used in specific circumstances. Plain radiographs are used if there is a history of trauma, if osteoporotic fractures are suspected in the elderly, or if spondyloarthropathies are suspected in younger patients. CT may be used for assessment of spondylolyses if MRI is contraindicated.

Further reading

* Royal College of Radiologists. *Making the Best Use of Clinical Radiology Services: Referral Guidelines*. 6th ed. London: Royal College of Radiologists; 2007.

42 e

Pectoralis minor does not form part of the rotator cuff. The supraspinatus, infraspinatus and teres minor tendons attach to the greater tuberosity. The subscapularis attaches to the lesser tuberosity. The supraspinatus is the most commonly injured tendon. Most tears occur in the so called 'critical zone' of the tendon which is a hypovascular area approximately 1–2 cm proximal to the tendon insertion. Tears appear as high signal on T2 weighted imaging, due to the presence of fluid. Normal tendons are of low signal intensity on all sequences.

43 d

A small anterior fat pad manifesting as a lucency immediately anterior to the distal humerus on the lateral radiograph may be seen in normal individuals. However elevation or increased size of the fat pad is abnormal and indicative of a joint effusion. A posterior fat pad is always abnormal, in the context of trauma, haemarthrosis secondary to an occult fracture is the likeliest explanation. In this patient's age group, the radial head is most likely to be injured; in children supracondylar fractures are more common. These injuries are often treated as radial head fractures even if a definite fracture line cannot be identified.

44 d

Rickets is due to failure of bone mineralisation due to vitamin D deficiency; the equivalent condition in adults is termed osteomalacia. Other features include delayed closing of fontanelles, softening of cranial vault and the so-called rachitic rosary (enlargement of cartilage at the costochondral junction).

45 c

PET-CT is a relatively new technique which combines the anatomical detail of CT with the functional ability of PET scanning. The PET component uses ^{18}FDG to determine glucose uptake. The effectiveness of the technique has led to its adoption in aiding surgical planning, radiation therapy and cancer staging. However it is expensive (the radioisotope is cyclotron produced) and carries a sizeable dose due to the fact that both components of the investigation involve radiation. The dose may be up to 25mSv (CXR dose is 0.02mSv).

46 b

In this age group with widening of the growth plate, a slipped upper femoral epiphysis must be considered. The frog leg view is able to identify the slipped epiphysis (which slips posteriorly relative to the femur) and also examine the other hip (up to 25% of cases are bilateral). Treatment is by internal fixation to prevent avascular necrosis.

47 e

In a trauma setting with a stable patient, CT is the most useful investigation for assessment of the solid organs as well as the GI tract and the bones. In an ideal situation a triple phase examination with images acquired pre-contrast, then in the arterial phase and in the venous phase post-i.v. contrast would be performed. In such circumstances, the spleen is the most commonly injured organ, followed by the liver.

48 a

This is the classic presentation of intussusception. Ultrasound is used to confirm the presence of a mass which characteristically has a 'target' like appearance due to hyperechoic fat being drawn into the mass and is the best first line investigation. AXR has been used in the past to demonstrate a soft tissue mass on the right with a paucity of bowel gas but has a low sensitivity. Air or hydrostatic contrast enema can be used as a therapeutic manoeuvre to reduce the intussusception; should this fail, surgery is required.

49 c

The presenting features of pain, swelling, tenderness, fever and a raised ESR can mimic infection. The additional feature of a soft tissue mass points towards the diagnosis. Ewing's sarcoma is derived from undifferentiated mesenchymal cells of the bone marrow or primitive neuroectodermal cells. It is a relatively common tumour which presents in the 5–15 year age range.

50 c

The likeliest diagnosis in a patient of this age is a metastasis from a lung carcinoma. A CXR would provide a simple and easy way to look for an underlying primary tumour. A bone scintigram could be performed to look for other bone metastases. Myeloma would be the likeliest primary bone tumour in this age group (however, much less common than metastasis) and if suspected (e.g. by virtue of Bence-Jones protein in the urine), a skeletal survey could be considered.

Chapter 8
Short answer questions (SAQs)

QUESTIONS

1   You make a request for a CT pulmonary angiogram in a patient with COPD and a suspected PE. What additional pieces of clinical information not relating to the patient's history or examination would be appropriate to include?

2   There are a number of patient related and non-patient related artefacts that can be confused with fracture lines on plain films of the extremities. Give three examples of such artefacts.

3   A routine CXR is performed in a 72-year-old woman pre-operatively for bypass surgery. No prior medical history is available.

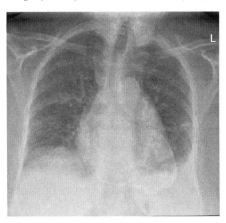 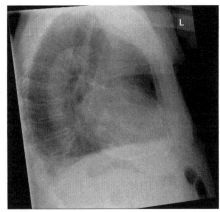

What is the main finding? List two possible causes for this.

4   A patient presents to the A&E department having suffered a sports-related neck injury. The patient is fully conscious with a GCS of 15. List three of the four factors needed to be present in order to clear the cervical spine clinically, without the need for plain films.

5   A 35-year-old man presents to the A&E department following a head injury. Give three factors in the history or on examination that would justify an urgent CT head examination.

6   A 46-year-old woman with known rheumatoid arthritis presents to her GP with shortness of breath. The GP requests a CXR for further investigation. List three CXR findings that have a known association with rheumatoid arthritis.

7   A 68-year-old man presents to his GP with haemoptysis. The GP requests a CXR:

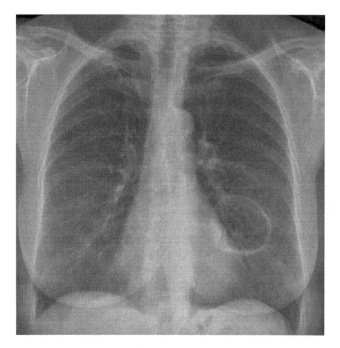

Describe the findings. List three possible differential diagnoses.

8   A neonate has three witnessed seizures. A CT head is requested and multiple areas of intracranial calcification are seen. The findings are thought to be secondary to a congenital infection. Name two possible causes.

9   A routine 20 week antenatal ultrasound reveals moderate hydrocephalus. List three causes of congenital hydrocephalus.

10 A 43-year-old man presents with recurrent haemoptysis. A CXR is requested and is reported as showing features of bronchiectasis within the left mid and lower zones. List three possible underlying aetiologies.

11 A patient is due to undergo an MRI examination. Give three absolute or relative contraindications to this procedure.

12 A 67-year-old man presents with increasing shortness of breath on minimal exertion. A CT chest is performed.

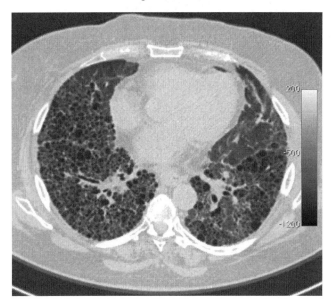

Image courtesy of Dr Vimal Raj (Leicester University Hospital).

What is the main finding? List two possible causes for this.

13 A hand X-ray shows diffuse osteopenia of the bones. List three possible causes.

14 A 47-year-old man presents with gradual onset of tiredness and new epigastric pain. A US is performed, blood tests are awaited. The liver, gallbladder and pancreas are normal in appearance; the spleen is noted to measure 17.1 cm in maximum length. Give three possible underlying causes for this appearance.

15 A CT chest is performed, which shows incidental enlargement of the right lobe of the thyroid, with retrosternal extension but no tracheal or oesophageal compression. List two possible causes.

16 A patient presents with shortness of breath. On examination there are bilateral rales and wheezing, predominantly in the mid zones. CXR shows bilateral mid and lower zone interstitial infiltrates. The FBC shows: Hb 13.7 g/dl, WCC 7.9 $\times 10^9$/l (normal = 4.3–10.8 $\times 10^9$/l), neutrophils 3.3 $\times 10^9$/l (2.5–7.5), eosinophils 1.1 $\times 10^9$/l (0.04–0.4). List three possible causes.

17 A pelvic X-ray is performed on a 47-year-old woman with bilateral hip pain.

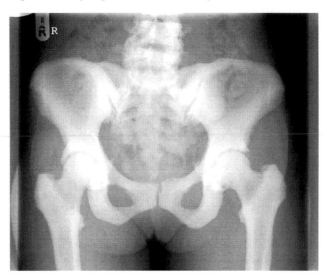

What is the main finding? List three possible causes for this.

18 A CXR shows the left hemidiaphragm to be raised above the right. There are no focal lesions, no evidence of lobar collapse, and the hilar regions are normal. List three possible causes.

19

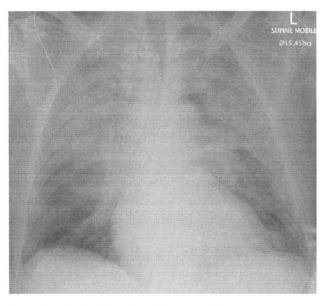

Describe the findings. List three possible causes.

20 A patient presents with a gradual onset of progressive dyspnoea, cough, fatigue, and weight loss. On examination there are inspiratory crepitations in the upper zones and the patient is noted to be clubbed. Lung function tests show a reduction in vital capacity and diffusion capacity. CXR shows fibrotic changes with loss of volume loss in the upper zones. List three possible underlying triggers that could be sought from questioning the patient.

21 A bone scintigram is performed and there is noted to be increased, asymmetrical uptake in the left knee. No history is readily available. List three possible causes.

22 A patient presents with gradual onset of right hip pain. A hip X-ray shows patchy sclerosis in the femoral head with flattening of the superior aspect of the femoral head, but preservation of the joint space. Avascular necrosis is suspected, list three potential cause of this.

23 A 19-year-old man presents to the A&E department with increasing shortness of breath. A CXR is performed:

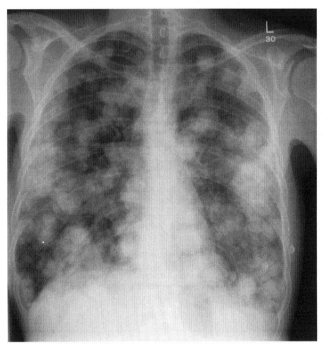

Describe the findings. What is the likely underlying diagnosis?

24 A 53-year-old man presents with vomiting, abdominal pain and bloating. On examination there are no signs of peritonism, but the bowel sounds are tinkling. AXR shows dilated loops of small bowel, measuring up to 5.5 cm, the large bowel is collapsed. Give three possible underlying causes.

25 A patient complains of chronic lower back pain, there is no history of trauma. The neurological examination is normal. X-rays of the lower lumbo-sacral spine show sclerosis and loss of joint space bilaterally within the sacro-iliac joints. List three possible causes.

26 History: a 43-year-old patient with gradually increasing shortness of breath on exercise.

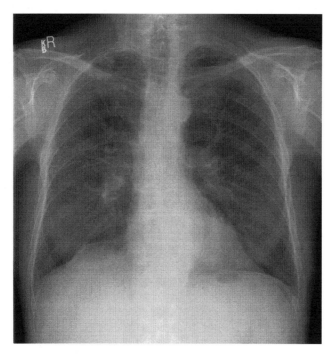

What is the main finding? List two possible causes for this.

27 A 43-year-old man presents to his GP with shortness of breath on exercise. A CXR is performed and shows interstitial fibrotic change within both upper zones. There is nil else of note. List three possible differential diagnoses.

28 A 54-year-old man presents with abdominal peritonism. List two plain film signs of abdominal perforation.

29 A patient presents with shortness of breath. There is noted to be asymmetrical, unilateral increased translucency of the left lung. List three possible causes.

30 A 73-year-old man presents with gradually increasing headache and drowsiness. A post-contrast CT head is performed.

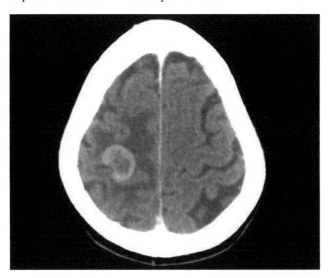

What is the main finding? List three possible causes for this.

ANSWERS

1   Additional useful information on a radiology request form includes:

- Serum creatinine level – iodinated i.v. contrast agents are potentially nephrotoxic.
- D-dimer level – if the level is normal it makes PE highly unlikely, if raised this would be consistent with a diagnosis of PE, but is a non-specific finding.
- Any prior reaction to iodinated contrast agents.
- Mode of transport – how can the patient travel to the department.
- MRSA or C. difficile status – important from an infection control point of view.
- Ward location – or if the patient is likely to be transferred to another ward.
- Contact details – your bleep or extension number if further clinical details or discussion is required.

2   Artefacts than can be confused with fracture lines include:

- External to the patient: clothing / bandages.
- Skin folds.
- Growth plates in paediatric patients.
- Harris ('growth arrest') lines.
- Sutures in the skull.
- Nutrient blood vessels.
- (Fracture 'fragments' may be mimicked by accessory ossicles, or normal anatomical variants.)

3   There is pericardial calcification, causes include:

- Prior pericarditis due to TB / rheumatic fever / viral infection.
- Post-cardiac surgery.
- Post traumatic.
- Uraemia.
- (apparent pericardial calcification: asbestos exposure, coronary artery calcification, LV aneurysm).

4   In order to 'clinically clear' the cervical spine, the patient needs to be fully alert and with the following criteria fulfilled:

- No posterior midline cervical spine tenderness.
- No evidence of intoxication.
- No painful distracting injury.
- No focal neurologic deficit on examination.

If there is any doubt cervical spine views should be obtained. At least three views are required: anterior-posterior (AP) view, open mouth odontoid ('PEG') view, and cross-table lateral view (which should include down to the inferior aspect and spinous process of the C7 vertebra). If necessary, a 'swimmer's' view can be used to enable better visualisation of the lower cervical vertebrae. Additional flexion and extension plain film views can be obtained to check for stability. If the plain film views are insufficient, CT can be performed; MRI is performed if a ligamentous injury is suspected.

Further reading
- Saddison D, Vanek VW, Racanelli JL. Clinical indications for cervical spine radiographs in alert trauma patients. *Am Surg.* 1991; **57(6)**: 366–9.
- Velmahos GC, Theodorou D, Tatevossian R, *et al.* Radiographic cervical spine evaluation in the alert asymptomatic blunt trauma victim: much ado about nothing. *J Trauma.* 1996; **40(5)**: 768–74.

5 NICE guidelines for CT head requests for adult patients presenting with a head injury.

Criteria for immediate request for CT scan of the head (adults)	Criteria for CT scan to be performed within 8 hours of injury*
GCS < 13 on initial assessment	Loss of consciousness or amnesia and one of
GCS < 15 at two hours after the injury	the following risk factors is present:
Suspected open or depressed skull fracture	• Age ≥65 years
Any sign of basal skull fracture	• Coagulopathy (history of bleeding, clotting
Post-traumatic seizure	disorder, current treatment with warfarin)
Focal neurological deficit	• Dangerous mechanism of injury:
> 1 episode of vomiting	• pedestrian struck by car
Amnesia for events > 30 minutes before	• occupant ejected from car
impact	• fall from a height > 1 m (or five stairs)

* Imaging should be performed immediately in these patients if they present eight hours or more after their injury.

Further reading
- NICE. *Head injury.* Guideline CG56: www.nice.org.uk/CG056.

6 CXR findings that have a known association with rheumatoid arthritis include:

- *Pleural effusion*: unilateral in 92%. Exudative due to raised protein levels, may also contain rheumatoid factor, LDH.
- *Pleural thickening:* usually bilateral.
- *Interstitial fibrosis:* lower lobe predominance.
- *Rheumatoid nodules:* identical to the subcutaneous nodules found in advanced RhA.
- *Caplan syndrome:* hypersensitivity reaction to dust particles in coal workers who have rheumatoid arthritis (rare!).
- *Bone abnormalities:* do not forget the bones on a CXR! Although unlikely to be associated with dyspnoea, the question asks, more generally, for associations with RhA. A classical finding in RhA is resorption of the distal ends of the clavicles, other features include erosion of the acromio-clavicular, shoulder, or sternoclavicular joints, and anklyosis of the vertebral bodies.
- *Others:* anti-rheumatoid drug side-effects: pericarditis / pericardial effusion.

Further reading
- Dahnert W, editor. *Radiology Review Manual.* 6th ed. Philadelphia, PA: Lippincott Williams & Wilkins; 2007.

7   There is a well defined mass adjacent to the left heart border, which is a cavitatory type lesion. There are no other lung lesions, no pleural effusions, the bones appear normal. The next appropriate imaging would be CT examination of the chest (*see* below), in this case the lesion was proven to be a primary SCC lung tumour.

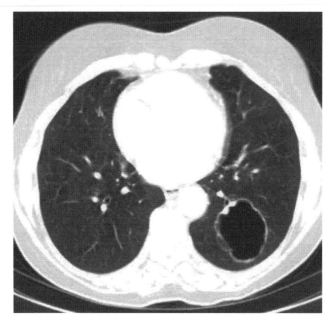

The 'surgical sieve' is often a good way to approach a list of differential diagnoses and is particularly useful in the case of cavitatory chest lesions. Causes include:

- *Tumours.*
  - Primary: particularly squamous cell lung cancer.
  - Secondary: metastases from tumours of squamous cell origin: cervical (women), oesophageal, nasopharyngeal.
- *Infection.*
  - Bacterial: staphylococcus aureus, Klebsiella.
  - Mycobacteria: tuberculosis.
  - Fungal: aspergillus.
- *Vasculitis.*
  - Wegener's granulomatosis.
  - Polyarteritis nodosum (rare).
  - Rheumatoid arthritis (Caplan syndrome).

8 Depending on the gestation time at which they occur, congenital central nervous system infections can result in serious malformations or tissue destruction. Intracranial calcification is common in the 'TORCH' infections:

- **TO**xoplasmosis.
- **R**ubella.
- **C**ytomegalovirus (most common).
- **H**erpes simplex.
- Others include: HIV infection, syphillis and varicella.

9 The causes of hydrocephalus can be broadly categorised as communicating (due to increased CSF production or reduced resorption at the level of the pacchionian granulation; typically symmetrical dilatation of all ventricles) and non-communicating (due to obstructive lesions at the intraventricular, foraminal, or aqueductal level, typically 'asymmetrical'). Neonatal causes of hydrocephalus include:

- *Communicating.*
  - Subarachnoid haemorrhage.
  - Meningitis.
  - Carcinomatous meningitis.
  - Venous infarct.
  - Choroid plexus tumour (increased production; rare).
- *Non-communicating.*
  - Aqueduct stenosis.
  - Dandy-Walker malformation.
  - Posterior fossa tumours.
  - Third ventricle tumours (e.g. ependymoma).

10 Bronchiectasis is defined as irreversible dilation of the bronchi (acute infections can cause dilatation, but this is reversible). Haemoptysis is a common presenting symptom. CT is very sensitive for the diagnosis: bronchi are seen to be of larger diameter than their accompanying vessel, do not taper down to a smaller size, have thickening of their walls and are seen within 1 cm of the pleural surface. Plain film can show tramlines, thickened end-on bronchi and atelectasis. Underlying causes fall into three broad categories:

- *Congenital.*
  - Cystic fibrosis.
  - Kartagener's syndrome (ciliary dysfunction).
  - Young's syndrome (similar to CF).
  - Inherited immunodeficiency syndromes (e.g. Common variable immunodeficiency).
- *Infection.*
  - Childhood infections: particularly measles and pertussis.
  - Tuberculosis.
  - Allergic broncho-pulmonary aspergillosis.

- *Post-obstructive.*
  - Children: inhaled foreign body.
  - Primary lung cancer.
  - Lymphadenopathy.

11 There are several absolute and relative contraindications to MRI. Most orthopaedic internal fixation devices are now MR-compatible, and it is only the older (> 20 years) devices that are likely to be ferromagnetic. If there is an appropriate history or high suspicion of metallic foreign bodies in the eye of a metal worker, plain films (or CT) of the orbits are obtained before scanning.

- *Absolute contraindications.*
  - Cardiac pacemakers.
  - Ferromagnetic implants.
  - Aneurysm clips (CNS).
  - Orbital metallic foreign body.
  - Cochlear implants.
- *Relative contraindications.*
  - Insulin pumps and nerve stimulators.
  - Non-ferromagnetic fixation devices (where the generation of heat can be a problem, particularly in MRI machines with higher magnetic field strengths).
  - Prosthetic heart valves (in high fields, if dehiscence is suspected).
  - Haemostatic clips (body).
  - Pregnancy (particularly first trimester).
  - (Claustrophobia.)

12 There is 'honeycombing' of the lung, whereby reticular fibrotic change summates to produce air-containing 'cysts' that are 0.5–2 cm in diameter. Causes include:

- Fibrotic lung disease: UIP, also known as cryptogenic fibrosing alveolitis (typical distribution: lower zones, subpleurally), NSIP, etc.
- Chronic extrinsic allergic alveolitis.
- Sarcoidosis (advanced, stage IV disease).
- Pneumoconioses: especially asbestosis.
- Collagen vascular disease-associated fibrosis: RhA, scleroderma.
- CF.
- Cystic bronchiectasis.
- Drug-related: nitrofurantoin, busulphan, bleomycin, cyclophosphamide.

13 Osteopenia is a decrease in the quantity of bone, which maintains its normal quality. This appears as an increased radiolucency on plain X-ray. Dual energy X-ray absorptiometry (DEXA) scans are used to differentiate normal / osteopenia / osteoporosis. Causes of diffuse osteopenia include:

- Primary osteoporosis.
- Secondary osteoporosis: malnutrition, calcium deficiency, protein deficiency, vitamin C deficiency, disuse / immobilisation.

- Endocrine: Cushing's, acromegaly, hyperparathyroidism, hyperthyroidism, Addison's, hypogonadism (Turner's syndrome), diabetes mellitus.
- Osteomalacia: vitamin D deficiency, renal osteodystrophy.
- Multiple myeloma.
- Drugs: heparin, phenytoin, methotrexate, corticosteroids, alcohol.
- Osteogenesis imperfect.
- Diffuse metastases (leukaemia).
- Mastocytosis.

14 The spleen measures approximately 11–13 cm on average and is located beneath the ninth to twelfth ribs. Spleen size varies with age, sex and height, but most accept splenomegaly as being > 13 cm. The causes of splenomegaly are divided by size: massive (> 20 cm), moderate, or mild, or by the pathological mechanism. Small spleen may be due to SCD (auto-infarcts), infarction, atrophy, polysplenia syndromes. Causes of splenomegaly include:

- Congestive: CCF, portal hypertension / cirrhosis, CF.
- Infective: CMV, malaria, Epstein-Barr virus.
- Cancer: leukaemia, lymphoma, myelofibrosis, metastases.
- Storage disorders: Gaucher disease, amyloidosis, sarcoid.
- Connective tissue disorders: RhA (Felty's syndrome), SLE.
- Haemolytic anaemias: hereditary spherocytosis.

15 The term 'toxic goitre' refers to goitre with hyperthyroidism. In general, goitre with normal hormone levels does not cause symptoms, aside from local pressure effects. Causes include:

- Normal variant: prominent pyramidal lobe present in 10%; enlarged during puberty.
- Iodine deficiency.
- Metastases to thyroid: most common primaries include breast, lung, kidney, melanoma, Hodgkin's disease.
- Pregnancy (increased physiological demands), also note post-partum thyroiditis.
- Thyroid amyloidosis.
- Hypothyroidism: Hashimoto's thyroiditis (can cause hyperthyroidism), congenital hypothyroidism, drug-induced (amiodarone).
- Hyperthyroid: Graves' disease, toxic multinodular goitre, de Quervain's thyroiditis, other causes of thyroiditis, thyroid cancer, thyroid lymphoma.

16 Eosinophilic lung disease is the presence of pulmonary infiltrates with an associated blood/tissue eosinophilia. Eosinophilia is defined as a peripheral eosinophil count > 0.44×10^9/l. Causes of eosinophilia and pneumonia include:

- Asthma.
- Loeffler's syndrome (acute eosinophilic pneumonia).
- Drugs: nitrofurantoin, sulfonamides, penicillin.
- Parasitic infections : ascariasis, schistosomiasis.
- Fungal infections: allergic broncho-pulmonany aspergillois.

- Vasculitis-related: Wegener's granulomatosis, Churg-Strauss, RhA, scleroderma, PAN, Sjögren's syndrome.

17 The striking feature is the diffuse osteosclerosis, with a diffuse increased density of the bones. *See* also the lateral thoracic spine radiograph in the same patient:

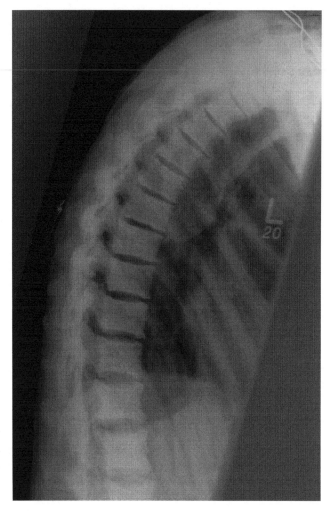

In this case the finding was due to fluorosis. Causes of osteosclerosis include:

- Fluorosis.
- Osteopetrosis.
- Diffuse osteosclerotic metastases (from prostate cancer, breast cancer, etc.).
- Mastocytosis.
- Myelofibrosis.
- Pyknodysostosis.
- Melorheostosis.
- Osteopoikilosis.

- Hyperparathyroidism.
- Sickle cell disease.
- Oxalosis.
- Paget's disease.
- Renal osteodystrophy.

18 The right diaphragm is normal approximately 1.5 cm superior to the left, they may be at a similar level, but elevation of the left above the right implies abnormality. Bilateral diaphragmatic elevation may be due to poor inspiratory effort, obesity, restrictive lung disease or neuromuscular disorders (motor neurone disease, myasthenia gravis), or bilateral phrenic nerve palsy (which can also be unilateral). In diaphragmatic paralysis, patients are often more short of breath lying flat, as the diaphragm normal plays an important role in supine respiration. This can be diagnosed dynamically by US or fluoroscopy: the diaphragm is seen to paradoxically move superiorly with inspiration (this can be accentuated by 'sniffing'). Causes of unilateral diaphragmatic elevation include:

- Phrenic nerve paralysis: primary lung tumour, malignant mediastinal tumour, iatrogenic (ligation of the nerve), idiopathic, secondary to polyneuritis.
- Reduced lung volume: atelectasis, post surgical (lobectomy), hypoplastic lung.
- Subphrenic abscess.
- Distended stomach / colon.
- Hepatic / splenic mass.
- Diaphragmatic hernia: Bochdalek or Morgagni types.
- Diaphragmatic eventration.
- Traumatic diaphragmatic rupture.
- Splinting of the diaphragm due to rib fracture / pleurisy.
- Hemiplegia: upper motor neurone lesion.
- Diaphragmatic tumour: mesothelioma, fibroma, lipoma, metastases.
- (Subpulmonic pleural effusion: gives the false impression of a raised diaphragm.)

19 There is diffuse bilateral alveolar airspace shadowing in a 'bat's wing' distribution. Although this is a supine film, the heart is at the upper limit of normal. There are no pleural effusions. Interstitial pulmonary oedema typically develops first (with Kerley B lines, etc.), when the fluid cannot be contained within the interstitial space, it passes into the alveoli to produce alveolar pulmonary oedema, as seen in this case. There are many causes of pulmonary oedema; broadly these can be divided into cardiogenic and non-cardiogenic.

- *Cardiogenic:*
  - Congestive cardiac failure.
  - Acute myocardial infarction with left ventricular failure.
  - Arrythymias.
  - Cardiac tamponade.

- *Non-cardiogenic:*
  - Fluid overload.
  - Neurogenic causes (SAH, seizures, head trauma).
  - Renal artery stenosis.
  - ARDS.
  - Polytrauma.
  - Drug abuse (cocaine, heroin).
  - Near drowning.
  - Altitude sickness.

20 Extrinsic allergic alveolitis is alveolar inflammation secondary to organic dusts inhaled either at the workplace, or through hobbies. It can be acute (within six hours of heavy exposure), subacute or chronic. It is thought to be a combination of a type III and type IV hypersensitivity reaction. Diagnosis is a combination of radiological findings, pulmonary function tests, demonstration of serum precipitins against the relevant antigen, and a positive provocation test. Triggers / syndromes include:

- Bagassosis: mouldy sugar cane.
- Bird-fancier's lung: pigeon keepers.
- Chemical worker's lung: manufacture of plastics, polyurethane foam, rubber.
- Crack lung: from cocaine smoking.
- Farmer's lung: working with mouldy hay.
- Humidifier / air conditioner lung.
- Malt worker's lung: malt dust.
- Maple bark disease: in saw mills.
- Miller's lung: dust contaminated grain.
- Mushroom worker's lung.
- Sequoiosis: redwood dust.
- Suberosis: mouldy cork dust.
- Wine grower's lung: mouldy grapes.

21 Hot spots on bone scans can be relatively non-specific and, depending on the clinical context, there are numerous potential causes, including:

- Fracture of the patella / distal femur / proximal tibia.
- Inflammatory arthritis, particularly Reiter's disease, inflammatory bowel associated arthritis, gout, pseudogout, or psoriatic arthritis. Rheumatoid arthritis is a possibility, but would be unusual.
- Metastases.
- Primary bone tumour: osteosarcoma, Ewing's sarcoma.
- Post-surgical joint replacement: 'hot' on BS up to one year.
- Infection: septic arthritis or osteomyelitis.
- Paget's disease.
- Soft tissue calcification causing uptake: myositis ossificans.
- Osgood-Schlatter's disease.
- (Degenerative osteoarthritis – although unusual to affect one large joint.)
- (Metabolic bone disease – but this would be expected to be diffuse.)

22 Causes of avascular necrosis include:

- Trauma: the blood supply to the femoral head means that, like the scaphoid bone, it is particularly prone to AVN following fracture of the femoral neck (transcervical and subcapital fractures).
- Excess alcohol intake: possibly due to fat embolism in chronic pancreatitis.
- Drugs: cortocsteroids, indomethacin, immunosuppressives.
- Haematopoetic disorders: sickle cell disease, haemophilia, polycythaemia rubra vera.
- Inflammatory: SLE, RhA, scleroderma.
- Post-infective.
- Bone replacement: Gaucher's disease.
- Fat embolism.
- Thermal injury.
- Post radiotherapy.
- Idiopathic: Perthe's disease.
- Post slipped capital femoral epiphysis.

23 There are multiple large, well-circumscribed lesions throughout both lungs. There is no pleural effusion, the bones appear normal. The findings are consistent with multiple lung metastases, their large nature means they can be appropriately described as 'cannon ball' metastases. Infection is a possibility, but far less likely given the appearances. Cannon ball metastases are classically found in renal cell carcinoma, but are also found in choriocarcinoma. In this young patient, the latter diagnosis was confirmed at testicular ultrasound.

24 Tinkling bowel sounds and the history imply bowel obstruction which is confirmed by the abdominal radiograph (small bowel of > 3 cm diameter is abnormal). It this case there is only small bowel obstruction described. Causes of small bowel obstruction include:

- Adhesions from previous surgery.
- Adhesions due to inflammatory strictures (Crohn's disease) or ischaemic strictures.
- Paralytic ileus: post-operative, or due to sepsis (e.g. appendicitis), or metabolic (e.g. hypokalaemia).
- Hernias (particularly inguinal hernias).
- Intussusception, common in children, usually due to a mass / lesion in adults.
- Volvulus.
- Foreign bodies (ingested; or a passed gallstone, 'gallstone ileus').
- Neoplasms, rare in small bowel.

25 Bilateral sacroilitis can be caused by:

- Ankylosing spondylitis.
- Inflammatory bowel-related arthropathy.
- Psoriatic arthropathy.
- Post-infective.

- Post-trauma.
- Degenerative osteoarthritis.
- (Osteitis condensans ilii: symmetric benign osteosclerosis of the portion of the iliac bones adjacent to the sacroiliac joints, particularly seen in young women post-partum.)

26 The most striking feature is bilateral enlargement of the pulmonary arteries, implying pulmonary hypertension (the upper limit of normal for the right and left pulmonary arteries is 1.5 cm). Causes of enlarged pulmonary arteries includes:

- Left-to-right shunts (when the ratio reaches 3:1).
- Hyperdynamic circulation: thyrotoxicosis, Beri-Beri, severe anaemia, Paget's disease.
- Pulmonary venous hypertension: mitral stenosis, LV failure.
- Idiopathic, primary pulmonary hypertension (typically young female patients).
- Chronic thrombo-embolic disease.
- Chronic lung disease, including COPD.
- Vasculitic disease, including PAN.

27 Certain conditions have a predilection for causing fibrotic change either within the upper or lower zones, however, there is some overlap.

- *Predominantly upper zone fibrosis:*
  - Berylliosis.
  - Radiotherapy induced.
  - Extrinsic allergic alveolitis.
  - Ankylosing spondylitis.
  - Sarcoidosis.
  - Tuberculosis (mneumonic: BREAST).
- *Predominantly lower zone fibrosis:*
  - Connective tissue disorders (e.g. RhA, scleroderma, dermatomyositis).
  - Drug induced (e.g. Nitrofurantoin, bleomycin, amiodarone).
  - Asbestosis.
  - Idiopathic pulmonary fibrosis (UIP: usual interstitial pneumonitis).
  - Aspiration.

28 The most sensitive test is an erect chest X-ray showing air under the diaphragm, which can show as little as 1 ml of free air. Signs on a supine or erect abdominal X-ray can be more subtle and harder to detect:

- Air-under the diaphragm: seen on erect CXR.
- Rigler's ('double wall') sign: caused by the presence of air on both sides of the bowel wall, usually requires >1000 ml free air.
- Football sign: large oval-shaped central radiolucency in the shape of an American football, may also have a well-defined linear opacity, the 'laces', which represents the air-outlined falciform ligament.

- Triangle sign: triangular pocket of air is seen between three loops of bowel; includes Doge's sign, when in Morrison's pouch.
- Falciform ligament clearly outlined.
- Ligamentum teres clearly outlined.
- Area of hyperlucency overlying the liver.
- Parahepatic free air.
- Air seen above the liver in a left lateral decubitus film (left-side down).

29 Causes of an asymmetrical, unilateral increased translucency of the lung include:

- Chest wall defect: unilateral mastectomy, and atrophy (polio) or absence of the pectoralis muscle (Poland's syndrome).
- Large airway obstruction with air trapping: inhaled foreign body, mucocoele, carcinoid, bronchial carcinoma.
- Small airways disease: MacLeod's (Swyer-James) syndrome, bronchioloitis obliterans.
- Decreased blood flow to the affected side: congenital pulmonary artery hypoplasia, PE.
- Compensatory hyperinflation following lobectomy.
- Congenital lobar emphysema.
- Asymmetrical emphysematous change (particularly bullous emphysema).
- Single lung transplant with emphysema of the native lung.
- Pneumothorax.
- (Patient rotation: gives the false impression of unilateral hyperlucency.)
- (Scoliosis: as above.)

30 The CT head shows a 4×3 cm ring-enhancing lesion in the right fronto-parietal region with surrounding oedema. In general, the low density centre is due to either avascularity (or low vascularity) or cystic degeneration. The 'ring-enhancing' edge is due to either hypervascular granulation tissue / hypervascular tumour capsule or increased permeability due to the breakdown of the blood-brain barrier (allowing leakage of contrast into the extracellular fluid space). Causes of ring-enhancing lesions include:

- Primary neoplasm: high grade glioma, lymphoma, leukaemia.
- Metastases.
- Infection: bacterial / tuberculous / fungal / parasitic abscess.
- Haemorrhagic-ischaemic lesion: resolving infarct, resolving haematoma, post surgical, thrombosed aneurysm.
- Demyelination: tumefactive multiple sclerosis.
- Drug-related.
- Radiation necrosis.

Chapter 9
Viva voce

QUESTIONS

1   What do you know about CT contrast agents? Do you know of any contra-indication, adverse-effects or cautions that apply for such agents?

2   Paediatric patients are preferentially imaged with US or MRI rather than CT. Why do you think this is so?

3   What do you know about the NHS breast screening programme? What happens when someone is recalled? Can you think of any disadvantages of the scheme?

4   A patient is brought in from a road traffic accident. What role do you think radiology has to play in the management of such patients? What modalities are most useful?

5   Radiation awareness and protection are key elements of radiology. What do you know about this and how can we help reduce the radiation exposure of patients?

6   What role do you think radiology plays in the detection and investigation of suspected non-accidental injury (NAI) in children? How are such children investigated? What findings would be particularly suspicious for NAI?

7   The majority of hospitals in the UK now use PACS (picture archiving communication system) and digital/computed radiography. What do you think are the main advantages of this? Can you think of any disadvantages?

8   What do you understand by the term 'functional' imaging in radiology? Do you know of any examples?

9   A 67-year-old man is found unconscious with a GCS of 8/15. Initial toxicology is normal and there is no collateral history available. What are the advantages of CT head imaging over MR imaging in the first instance? What additional information can MR head imaging provide?

10 A patient needs a chest X-ray but is concerned that it involves radiation, how would you explain the radiation involved and the risks entailed, using simple terms?

11 What do you understand by the term 'skills mix'? How do you think it applies to radiology? How do you think government targets relate to this? What are the key areas of healthcare and radiology that can benefit from this?

12 What do you know about teleradiology / radiology outsourcing? Discuss any relevant advantages / disadvantages of teleradiology. How do you see the future of this?

13 If there is a critical, urgent, or unexpected significant radiological finding, who is responsible for this result? How should the result be communicated?

14 There are particular concerns with using radiation in patients who are pregnant. What controls are in place for such patients? How can dose be limited for these patients? How should diagnostic practice be adapted?

15 Do you think it is necessary for a hospital to have 24-hour coverage by a radiologist? Why? If yes, is teleradiology the answer? What considerations would need to be taken into account if implementing such 24-hour cover?

ANSWERS

1

CT contrast agents can be given orally, rectally, or intravenously. Some indications for CT imaging do not require contrast administration (e.g. CT abdomen / pelvis for renal colic, where stones need to be detected), others cannot be performed without contrast media (e.g. CT-pulmonary angiogram).

The positive oral contrast agent that is typically used is dilute Gastrografin®; if the large bowel needs to be opacified then a 'long oral' preparation is necessary (administering the contrast 48 hours before scanning). Water can be used as a 'negative contrast agent', which is particularly useful when imaging the upper GI tract, e.g. pancreatic imaging. There are no real contra-indications for oral agents, providing the patient is safely able to swallow liquids, but they are unlikely to be tolerated in small bowel obstruction (fluid-filled loops mean contrast is less of a necessity regardless).

Intravenous contrast agents are iodine based and have the potential for causing two types of complications: acute renal failure and an anaphylactoid reaction to the iodinated-agent. Non-ionic, low-osmolar agents are 5–10× safer than the older high osmolar ionic agents. 'Anaphylactoid' reactions are similar to anaphylactic reactions but are not true hypersensitive reactions and do not involve IgE. They do not require pre-sensitisation and can occur with as little as 1 ml of contrast medium; subsequent exposures do not necessarily result in the same reaction. The incidence of major reactions is rare: incidence of 'serious' reactions is 0.04% and of 'life-threatening' reactions is 0.004%. There is an increased risk of such reactions if there is a history of atopy, asthma, B-blocker usage (all increase the risk ×3), cardiac disease (×5), age > 50 years (×2) and previous allergic reaction to iodine or shellfish (×10). There is no conclusive evidence that pre-medication with steroids is of benefit.

The risk of iodinated contrast agents causing nephrotoxicity is increased if pre-existing renal impairment is present (particularly with a creatinine > 133 μmol/L). Other factors that increase risk include: metformin use, NSAID use, and type-2 diabetes mellitus. Ensuring adequate hydration is recommended. Many radiology departments recommend stopping metformin before administration and for 48 hours thereafter, however, recent RCR guidelines suggest that if the renal function is normal and a standard volume of contrast is to be administered (< 100 mls), such precautions are unnecessary.

Further reading

- RCR. *Standards for iodinated intravascular contrast agent administration to adult patients 2005*. RCR: London; updated 2009.
- Kessel D, Robertson I, editors. *Interventional Radiology: a survival guide*. 2nd ed. London: Elsevier, Churchill-Livingstone; 2005: 12–14.

2

Children are particularly at risk from radiation exposure because:

- The effects of radiation are greatest when growth is fastest, especially in the foetal period (organogenesis can be affected), and during infancy and childhood (increased risk of carcinogenesis).

- Children have a longer life expectancy in which to manifest the harmful effects of radiation. For instance, if there is increased risk of developing lymphoma 20–30 years post-exposure, this is obviously less of a concerned in a patient > 75 yrs old.
- Children's organs are more radiosensitive compared to adults.
- Children's organs receive a higher dose per examination compared to adults.
- There is the potential for multiple non-diagnostic exposures in an unco-operative child.
- Failure to modify pre-set 'adult' parameters (e.g. CT) when children are scanned will increase their dose.

Additional discussion of the risks of radiation including 'stochastic' and 'deterministic' effects may be appropriate. Deterministic effects are 'all-or-nothing' such as fibrosis or radiation burns, which only occur above a certain threshold; this is less relevant to diagnostic procedures, but may be encountered with radiotherapy regimes. Stochastic effects as based on the fact that all radiation is considered harmful, and that there is an accumulation of risk of future cancer development with further exposures.

Further reading
- Kuhn JP, Slovis TL, Haller JO, editors. *Caffey's Pediatric Diagnostic Imaging*. 10th ed. St Louis, MO: Mosby; 2003: vol 1, section 1, 1–12.
- Brenner D, Elliston C, Hall E, *et al*. Estimated risks of radiation-induced fatal cancer from pediatric CT. *AJR*. 2001; **176**: 289–96.

3

The NHS National Breast Screening Programme was introduced in England and Wales in 1988, following recommendations made in the Forrest report. Initially women aged 50–64 years were invited for breast screening by mammography every three years, however, it was not until 1995 that all eligible women were invited for screening. Recently this age range has been expanded to those aged 50–70 inclusive, and the Government is planning to further increase the breast screening programme to cover women aged 47–73 by the year 2012. Patients are invited to return at three-yearly intervals. Two views are obtained as standard: the cranio-caudal view (superior-inferior view) and the medial-lateral oblique (MLO) view – a lateral view with angulation. Patients with a suspicious lesion are recalled for further testing, where repeat views are obtained, often with 'compression' views, an ultrasound performed and, if deemed necessary, a biopsy taken. Biopsies can be performed under US guidance (if visible by US), or stereotactically, using X-ray guidance.

The aim of screening is to detect breast cancer at an earlier, potentially curable stage. The current detection rate is approximately six cancers per 1000 women screened. Potential disadvantages include the anxiety caused by recalling patients and harm from invasive testing if the results ultimately turn out to be negative. Another potential disadvantage is false-reassurance, for instance, it may be that some women think they do not need to regularly examine their breasts for lumps if their last screening test was normal. Separate screening protocols are in place for high risk patients, e.g. those who received mantle radiotherapy for non-Hodgkin's lymphoma, those with a strong family history, or BRCA gene carriers.

Further reading
- Forrest APM. *Breast cancer screening: report to the health ministers of England, Wales, Scotland and Northern Ireland*. London: HMSO; 1986.
- NHS. *Quality assurance guidelines for breast screening radiology*. NHSBSP publication 59; January 2005.

4

If the patient is haemodynamically unstable with internal injuries then an emergency laparotomy should be performed immediately. In the more stable patient, radiological investigations can be used to direct management.

CXR: useful to diagnose pneumothoraces, rib fractures, haemothorax, and can provide an indication of thoracic aortic transection (widened mediastinum). If a tension pneumothorax is suspected treatment should be performed immediately. An erect chest X-ray is often not possible in the trauma setting to help diagnose free intra-abdominal air.

Axial skeleton and limb films: useful for limb fractures, pelvic fractures and cervical / thoracic / lumbo-sacral fractures.

Ultrasound: recently, emergency department doctors have been trained in basic ultrasound, and the use of focused US in the trauma situation has almost become an extension of the physical examination: the assessment of 'circulation'. The so called 'FAST' (focused assessment with sonography for trauma) scan is a US scan directed at looking for pericardial fluid indicative of tamponade, or identifying free intraperitoneal fluid, which in the context of trauma is likely to be due to haemorrhage. This is quick to perform and has largely replaced the previously used 'diagnostic peritoneal lavage'.

CT: this forms the mainstay of diagnostic investigation in the trauma patient. More accurate information can be provided on the presence and extent of fractures, pneumothoraces, haemothorax, diaphragmatic rupture, free intraperitoneal fluid, and organ damage. 'Triple' phase imaging is performed, i.e. three CTs: without i.v. contrast medium, in the arterial phase post-contrast administration, and in the portal phase post-contrast. An additional delayed series may be required if renal trauma is suspected, in order to look at the collecting systems. The pre-contrast scan is useful for showing haemorrhage (acutely blood is seen as bright on CT), the arterial phase is useful for showing the source of bleeding.

Angiography / interventional radiology: in certain circumstances radiology can be used for treatment. If a vascular injury is confirmed or suspected, angiography can aid diagnosis and can potentially be used to treat points of bleeding: either by embolisation (e.g. bleeds from branch vessels or organs) or by stent placement (e.g. aortic transection).

5

The Ionising Radiation (Medical Exposure) regulations (IR(ME)R) lay down basic measures for the health protection of individuals against the dangers of ionising radiation in relation to medical exposure. There are no 'set limits' for patient exposure as it is a risk / benefit pay off, but every examination must be justified and contribute to patient management. The practitioner (usually a radiographer for simple plain film requests, or radiologist for CT or high exposure procedures) accepts the referral as justified, however, the referrer has a responsibility to provide sufficient, relevant and correct medical data. If it is necessary to use a test that involves ionising radiation then satisfactory image quality (not necessarily the most optimal image) should be obtained using radiation exposures that conform to the principle of ALARP (as low as reasonably practicable). Ways to reduce / limit radiation exposure include:

- Avoid unnecessary examinations.
- Using modalities with no radiation dose to answer the clinical question (US, MRI), or using the imaging modality / technique that gives the lowest dose.
- Obtaining image quality that is adequate to answer the clinical question, rather than striving for the most optimal images – this applies particularly to CT.
- Use of techniques such as digital radiographs, where post-processing can alter contrast levels, rather than necessitating repeat views.
- Lead shielding to avoid exposing areas not relevant to the clinical problem, examples include gonad shielding and also using collimation of the X-ray beam.
- Correct patient positioning, which enables appropriate centring of the beam.
- Minimise the number of exposures per examination: some tests require multiple views, e.g. two views for most suspected fractures, but the routine use of a lateral chest radiograph, or comparison views of the 'normal' limb is inappropriate, except in agreed circumstances.
- Special consideration should be given when imaging high risk groups such as pregnant woman and children, discussion with a senior radiologist would be appropriate.

6

Imaging studies are often critical in the assessment of the injured infant and young child and they commonly provide support for allegations of child abuse. Although skeletal injuries rarely pose a threat to the life of the abused child, they are often the strongest radiologic indicators of NAI. Especially in infants and very young children with NAI, where externally visible injuries are often absent, imaging studies are sometimes the first indication of abuse. The majority of physically abused children will present in one of three ways in the radiology department:

- Referred for imaging with a high clinical suspicion of NAI.
- A radiological test reveals lesions not consistent with the clinical history.
- Incidental findings on a radiological exam performed for another reason.

A skeletal survey is a series of plain X-ray films which images the entire skeleton / anatomical regions for signs of injury. It reveals information on the nature, location and chronicity of injury, and can provide objective evidence of abuse in child protection cases or criminal proceedings. The British Society of Paediatric Radiology state that a skeletal survey for NAI is indicated if there is suspected physical abuse in infants / young children (occult injury is rare in those > 3 years), or in siblings (< 3 years) of children with proven NAI. The skeletal survey includes 20 standard views; additional views are taken if required.

- *Standard views (total = 20)*:
  - AP chest.
  - AXR (to include pelvis and hips).
  - Lateral C-spine.

- Lateral thoraco / lumbar spine.
- Single AP and lateral skull.
- Bilateral views of: humeri, forearms, femurs, tibias/fibulas, hands, feet.
- Bilateral oblique rib views.
- *Supplemental views:*
  - Towne's (if suspected occipital injury).
  - Coned views of the relevant joint (metaphyseal injury).
  - Lateral views of a relevant long bone (diaphyseal fracture).
  - CT head if neurological signs / drowsiness present, or if there is suspicion of a subdural haematoma.

Although they are less-specific for NAI (occurring frequently in accidental injury), diaphyseal fractures occur 4× more frequently than the more NAI-characteristic metaphyseal fractures. A key diagnostic feature of NAI is the presence of multiple fractures of differing ages.

Fractures with high specificity for NAI	Fractures with moderate specificity for NAI	Fractures with low specificity for NAI (but occur frequently)
Outer third clavicle	Multiple fractures	Middle third clavicle
Metaphyseal	Fractures of differing ages	Greenstick fracture radius
Posterior ribs	Spiral fractures of humerus	Linear parietal bone fracture
Scapula	Digital injury in non-mobile child	Spiral tibial fracture in a mobile child
Spinous processes		Single diaphyseal fractures
Sternal		
Depressed occipital fracture		

If neurological signs are present, or head injury is suspected, a CT head or MRI head should be performed. Subdural haematomas (SDH) are the most common intracranial finding in NAI (accidental causes of SDH in this age group are rare). Features that strongly correlate SDHs to NAI are: associated presence of retinal haemorrhage (implying shaking injury), bilateral SDHs, SDHs of differing ages, and SDH without an underlying fracture (shaking).

Bone scintigraphy can be used in the work-up of NAI. The radiation dose is higher, but they have an increased sensitivity, particularly for evaluation of rib and long bone abnormalities. However, specificity is low as any fracture (even accidental) will show increased uptake. Bone scans are not accurate for the evaluation of metaphyseal injuries or skull fractures due to the increased activity in the growth plates and sutures, respectively. Plain film is better at determining fractures of different ages as the healing processes have different radiographic features; old fractures may have no activity on scintigraphy.

Further reading
- British Society of Paediatric Radiology: www.bspr.org.uk/nai.htm.
- Swinson S, Tapp M, Brindley R, *et al*. An audit of skeletal surveys for suspected non-accidental injury following publication of the British Society of Paediatric Radiology guidelines. *Clin Radiol*. 2008; **63(6)**: 651–6.

7

The use of digital / computed radiography to acquire images means that it is no longer necessary to deal with complicated film developing equipment and processes, nor to use expensive and toxic chemicals. In turn this reduces the time taken to perform an image and increases patient through-put. With digital radiography it is also less likely that a non-diagnostic image will be produced (i.e. over- or under-exposed) as post processing means the image contrast can be changed; this theoretically reduces unnecessarily repeated patient radiation exposure. Conversely, a potential disadvantage of this system is that overexposures may be masked; radiographers need to be aware of this and calibration is important. Other advantages specifically related to the PACS system are listed below.

- *Potential advantages:*
  - Following acquisition, the image cannot be lost, stolen, or misfiled. This means studies will not need to be repeated, clinical decisions not deferred, and patient appointments will not need to be cancelled on the basis of films being unavailable.
  - There is no longer a need for film storage rooms, nor 'dark' rooms for film processing, making more space available within the hospital.
  - Old studies can be easily retrieved in chronological order, for direct comparison.
  - Images can be viewed anywhere in the hospital and even outside. This makes images more likely to be reported and has been proven to reduce the time in which it takes for reports to be made available.
  - 'Teleradiology' is possible: reporters can view the images remotely, or images can be sent to colleagues at tertiary referral centres anywhere in the world for a specialist opinion.
  - Image can be viewed simultaneously, thus an ITU doctor can discuss an image with a radiologist without needing to leave the department.
  - Post-processing by altering contrast width and level allows both soft tissue and bony structures to be easily seen on a single exposure (e.g. on a CXR). Windowing may also make subtle findings, such as minimally displaced fractures, more apparent.
- *Potential disadvantages:*
  - The initial installation of fully integrate PACS systems hospital-wide is expensive, however, the future healthcare savings of the system would be expected to cover this initial outlay.
  - As with any IT-based system, PACS has the potential for a total system failure. Daily data backup should be routine to try and guard against this.
  - The clinician needs basic computer literacy in order to operate the workstations; this is not expected to be a problem for the current generation of junior doctors.
  - Initial basic training on the PACS is necessary which may be time consuming.
  - 'Over-windowing' has the potential to 'introduce' artefacts (increased noise) into the image, which may lead to misinterpretation.

Further reading
- Strickland, N. Current topic: PACS (picture archiving and communication systems): filmless radiology. *Arch Dis Child*. 2000; **83**: 82–6.

8

Traditionally, imaging modalities have been used to provide 'static' images, which provide anatomical, rather than functional information. 'Functional' imaging is a broad term, essentially relating to any imaging modality / technique that provides *in vivo* functional information for the region of the body scanned. With current imaging modalities being close to the best resolution obtainable, future advances in imaging are likely to be via functional imaging techniques or contrast agents.

In current practice, nuclear medicine tests provide functional information, examples include V/Q scanning, renal imaging, and PET scanning. Ultrasound can provide information on blood flow using the Doppler effect. Functional MRI techniques that are commonly used include diffusion weighted-imaging and spectroscopy, additionally dynamic-contrast enhanced techniques are being more widely used (particularly for breast cancer) and can provide information on tumours, based on rapid wash-in and wash-out of the contrast agent. The combination of different modalities can help overcome the disadvantages and limitations of each individual modality. PET-CT is a successful example of multimodal imaging, combining the excellent anatomical resolution of CT with the functional imaging provided by PET scanning.

Research is being undertaken on targeted imaging agents. Such macromolecules can incorporate targeting ligands, such as antibodies to potential allow highly specific imaging and even delivery of drug payloads directly to tumours. Although very much at the development stage, MRI agents currently show the most promise in this field.

9

CT is readily available in most hospitals, whereas access to MRI is often more limited, particularly out of hours. Advantages of CT in the acute situation described include:

- Better at showing acute haemorrhage if a haemorrhagic stroke is suspected, i.e. subarachnoid haemorrhage, subdural haematoma, extradural haematoma, parenchymal haemorrhage.
- Quick scan time. If the patient is unable to remain still for a prolonged period, the MR images are likely to be non-diagnostic, this is much less of a problem with CT, where images are acquired in a matter of seconds.
- Better at showing potential skull fractures, as trauma is a possibility.
- No real contraindications (*cf* MRI if the patient is known to have a pacemaker, or metal work *in situ*).

In the less acute situation, MRI can offer additional information including:

- Better soft tissue definition between grey and white matter.
- Better at showing subtle but potential devastating changes of 'diffuse axonal injury' from rapid acceleration / deceleration type injuries.
- Better able to different acute from chronic ischaemia.
- Better able to demonstrate old haemorrhage / haematoma.
- (No ionising radiation – more important if recurrent follow up imaging is required and in younger patients).

10

Internet resources mean patients are more informed than ever before and want to know the risks and benefits of procedures and investigations that are scheduled. Media coverage has further heightened patient awareness of radiation exposure from medical investigations and all doctors requesting radiation-involving investigations should have adequate knowledge of the relevant radiation doses. In the UK the average background radiation dose is 2.23 mSv per year (radon within the ground is the highest contributor at 59%), this rises to 2.64 mSv per year if medical exposures are taken into account. In the mentioned scenario, you essentially need to 'consent' the patient for having the investigation, one of the basic tenets of consent is presenting information using descriptions/language that the patient can understand and relate to. Topics that patients can relate to include background radiation and radiation received from airline flights; the radiation received from a standard CXR is approximately the same as that received from a return flight from London to Spain, an extremity X-ray is similar to that of a single flight from London to Paris.

Investigation	Effective dose (mSv)	Equivalent UK-average background radiation time (equivalent dose from a commercial flight is given, where appropriate)
Extremity X-ray	0.001	< 1 day (flight to Paris)
Chest X-ray	0.02	3 days (return flight to Spain)
Mammography	0.7	100 days
Abdominal X-ray	1	150 days
IVU	3	16 months
CT head	2	11 months
CT chest	5.8	2.7 years
CT chest, abdomen, pelvis	9.9	4.5 years
^{99m}Tc-MDP bone scan (740 MBq injected)	4.2	2 years

Another method to describe investigations with a higher radiation dose is to quote the equivalent number of chest X-rays: an AXR has approximately 50× the radiation dose of a CXR, CT radiation is considerably more. There is no such thing as a 'safe' radiation dose, but there is the diagnostic and potential treatment benefit to take into consideration; as such IR(ME)R regulations do not list 'dose limits' for patients (only for healthcare workers, family members, or the general public). As with any medical procedure there is a risk/benefit ratio to consider and the benefit of diagnosis and potential treatment options should outweigh the risks from the radiation exposure – which is also considered by the radiologist who accepts or declines the initial request. An example of this is performing a CT to exclude appendicitis in a borderline case, which may save the patient an unnecessary operation and the subsequent anaesthetic and operative risks, along with cosmetic considerations.

Further reading
* The Ionising Radiation (Medical Exposure) Regulations 2000: www.opsi.gov.uk/si2000/20001059.htm.

11

The 'skills mix' is a relatively new concept in UK healthcare, proposed by the government in order to maximise healthcare provision and address imbalances in the physician / nurse ratios that may exist in different regions. It is a relatively broad term which can refer to the mix of staff in the workforce, or changes in the demarcation of roles. Skill-mix changes may involve enhancement of skills among a particular staff group, sharing of duties amongst different groups, and innovation in new or existing staff roles. It aims to define multidisciplinary teams not by profession, but by the skills and competencies of the healthcare individuals in order to best meet the patient's needs. It mainly relates to skill-mix changes between physicians and nurses, however, in radiology, the 'skills mix' predominantly relates to the roles of radiologists and radiographers.

The relative shortage of radiographers, radiologists and oncologists has led to pressure for more staff, more equipment and the sharing of key skills / roles. In 1999, a Downing Street cancer summit identified three discrete service areas for service and infrastructure investment plans:

- Breast screening (and the expansion of the programme).
- Therapeutic radiology.
- Diagnostic radiology (including ultrasonography).

Thus, the 'skills mix' programme, which initially focused on breast screening, has been extended to encompass other areas of clinical imaging and radiotherapy. Furthermore, there are a number of government led goals and targets for the provisional of healthcare in general and cancer care in particular. Radiology is at the forefront of many of these targets, because imaging and image-guided biopsy is an essential part of the diagnostic pathway. The following NHS Cancer Plan waiting time targets have now been implemented:

- *2-week target*: from date of referral by GP to first review by a relevant specialist.
- *31-day target*: interval from diagnosis to first definitive treatment for cancer.
- *62-day target*: interval from urgent GP referral to first definitive treatment.
- *(Non-cancer related: 18-week target*: from the time patients are referred to the start of their hospital treatment.)

Potential pitfalls or disadvantages of the skills-mix programmes include the following:

- Compromised training of junior doctors.
- Inadequately defined lines of responsibility.
- Inter-professional rivalry.
- Loss of flexibility.
- Fragmentation of care.

Further reading
- www.dh.gov.uk/prod_consum_dh/groups/dh_digitalassets/@dh/@en/documents/digitalasset/dh_4061260.pdf.
- www.rcr.ac.uk/docs/radiology/pdf/Teamworking.pdf.
- Buchan J, Ball J, O'May F. If changing skill-mix is the answer, what is the question? *J Health Serv Res Policy*. 2001; **6(4)**: 233–8.

12

The RCR defines teleradiology as 'the electronic transmission of radiographic images from one geographical location to another for the purposes of interpretation and consultation'. Older systems were slow and capable of dealing with only small data sets, however, it is now possible for large data sets to be transmitted without loss of data. Additionally, the development of secure networks allows for safe data transfer.

- *Potential advantages of teleradiology:*
    - Rapid transmission of images via high-speed connections to major tertiary centres for evaluation and advice, regardless of distance. This is of benefit to DGHs, and is of particular value to hospitals in remote locations.
    - May avoid unnecessary transfer of patients to tertiary referral centres if it is deemed the care can be provided locally.
    - May avoid repeat examinations if the patient is transferred to a tertiary centre.
    - Case conferences can occur between clinical radiologists and clinicians from other hospitals.
    - Out-of-hours cover for image reporting can be provided remotely if there is inadequate staff numbers locally to provide 24-hour cover. This can also be exploited across time zones, with bilateral agreements between hospitals to provide out of hours cover (e.g. between English and Australian hospitals).
    - Images can be transferred to the home of the radiologist which offers better access to expert opinion and may have a beneficial effect on the work/life balance. This also potentially provides better support for junior radiologists and also junior clinicians (with senior members of their own team).
    - Can be used for improved medical education when teleradiology is used for tutorials and case presentations.
    - Private outsourcing can be used to report studies remotely to clear backlogs or to provide a routine service and reduce waiting lists where supply cannot be met locally (e.g. MRI).
    - Outsourcing to centres with more radiologists means that higher quality control such as compulsory double reading can theoretically be achieved.
    - As a purely economic model, teleradiology places the in-hospital radiologist in direct competition with all other worldwide suppliers. This competition will drive down costs, which means healthcare providers will have excess money to spend on other goods and services.
- *Potential disadvantages of teleradiology:*
    - There are several potential legal issues in using teleradiology. These are predominantly applicable to the provision of a teleradiology service from outside national boundaries. The registration of the reporting radiologist must be recognised by the local governing body.
    - Radiologists in other countries will not undergo local revalidation and it may be difficult to establish if they have appropriate continuing medical education to maintain training for the tasks to be undertaken.
    - There are numerous potential legal issues that may arise from outsourcing of work. The NHS Trust ultimately bears responsibility for patient care and for the actions of doctors it employs. However, for contracts between Trusts

and teleradiology suppliers, liability of the supplier of the service and the reporting radiologist need to be clearly defined.

- The teleradiology service must be robust enough to ensure patient confidentiality and comply with data protection legislation.
- The principles of ALARP need to be applied in order to limit patient radiation dose. If scan protocols are defined by the teleradiology service, there is a risk that higher dose protocols may be used in all cases to improve scan quality, irrespective of the clinical indication.
- Providers of a teleradiology service would expect to practice in the same way as they would within their own population, which may be different to UK departments. Additional investigations may be requested which may further pressurise services and increase the population radiation dose.
- An important component of radiology is communication with the referring clinician, not just via the written report but also through further dialogue. If reporting examinations remotely, this clinical contact between the referring clinicians is substantially reduced.
- Formal and informal discussions between radiologist and clinician often result in a change of the diagnosis, by placing the case in the appropriate clinical context, e.g. multidisciplinary meetings, telephone, bleep, intranet, corridor consultations, etc. Such opportunities are greatly diminished with teleradiology.
- If there is an unexpected or urgent finding, urgent communication channels need to be in place to ensure reports are rapidly conveyed to the clinician responsible for the patient; this may be more difficult with teleradiology.
- Linguistic problems may arise, particularly if English is not the first language of the reporter. Standardisation may be necessary to ensure that things are not 'lost in translation'. This is also true for the use of abbreviations in reports or in requests, for instance TOF means 'tracheo-oesophageal fistula' in the UK and 'tetralogy of fallot' in the USA.
- It is often important to compare images to prior relevant studies, the teleradiology reporting service may not have such access to prior investigations and reports as a radiologist working in the primary department.
- 'Hands-on' radiology cannot be provided (e.g. ultrasound, fluoroscopy studies, image-guided interventions), which may be a problem if a cross-cover out of hours service is being provided.
- Transfer of all images in, for instance, a single subspecialist area such as musculo-skeletal or neuroradiology, will result in de-skilling of the local radiologists in these areas.
- Local disease prevalence may affect the interpretation by reporting radiologists, e.g. the interpretation of multiple pulmonary nodules is likely to be different in the UK than in India or even the USA.

Further reading

- www.rcr.ac.uk/publications.aspx?PageID=310&PublicationID=195
- http://content.nejm.org/cgi/reprint/354/7/662.pdf

13

Ultimately the clinician who requested the test and who is responsible for the care of the patient is responsible for the test result, however, there is now an acknowledgement that the reporting radiologist has an increasingly responsible role in communicating an important abnormal result. In the USA, failure to communicate a result is the fourth commonest cause for litigation against radiologists. The 2004 Department of Health publication 'Manual of cancer measures' emphasised the need for a system for reporting new or unsuspected cancers 'over and above the normal reporting mechanisms'. The RCR has recently provided its own guidance on such issues. More recently, the NHS National Patient Safety Agency (Safer Practice Notice 16) recommended that radiology departments and radiologists ensure that critical findings are emphasised in reports, are obvious, and that the degree of urgency for action is clear. Also 'safety net' procedures should be in place (e.g. copying reports to GPs or cancer MDTs) and regular audits of the system should be undertaken.

Methods of communication include radiographer 'red dots', phoning the result through to the ward or to the clinical team, emails, dedicated 'alert' systems, and faxing reports to the GP or the appropriate clinic. There has been a natural reluctance amongst UK radiologists to assume responsibility for ensuring that clinicians receive, read, and act upon abnormal reports; this may be difficult practically and some argue that the person requesting a test / investigation is responsible for obtaining and acting upon the result. However, many departments already have mechanisms in place for expediting appropriate referral for unsuspected cancers. Moreover, effective communication of urgent information is essential for safe patient care and to ensure that harm does not result from imaging findings being overlooked despite being correctly reported. The RCR defines the following types report urgency:

- Critical findings – emergency action is required as soon as possible.
- Urgent findings – medical evaluation is required within 24 hours.
- Significant unexpected findings – the radiologist has concerns the findings are significant and they will be unexpected.

'Critical' findings necessitate immediate communication with the clinical team, the most appropriate means is likely to be via telephone / bleep systems. However, for the other two categories there are various potential methods of communication available and the third category is by its nature subjective. The RCR recommends that each department should define and develop policies for communication of important clinical findings. However, this should not replace the responsibility of each referrer to read the result of investigations they request, but rather, is a safety net for highlighting significant findings. There is also acknowledgement that trusts may need to invest in IT systems for more reliable methods to be put in place.

Further reading
- RCR. *Standards for the communication of critical, urgent and unexpected significant radiological findings*. London: RCR; 2008.
- NHS National Patient Safety Agency. Safer Practice Notice 16. *Early identification of failure to act on radiological imaging reports*. London: NPSA; 2007.

14

There are two types of radiation-induced effects and both are relevant to the unborn foetus.

1   Deterministic effects, resulting from damage to a number of cells, from which there is a dose threshold which has to be exceeded before effects are manifest. Examples include foetal death, malformation, growth retardation and abnormal brain development leading to mental retardation.
2   Stochastic effects, originate from damage to single cells. There is no dose threshold, but the risk increases as dose increases (e.g. developing a radiation-induced cancer).

When pregnancy is established: consideration needs to be given to other investigations which do not involve ionising radiation (ultrasound, MRI). Examples include doing bilateral leg lower limb venous scans to look for a DVT in the work-up of suspected PE. Although the safety of MRI is not fully established (particularly in the first trimester), it is still preferable to procedures which directly irradiate the foetus.

When pregnancy status is not known: for all examinations where the X-ray beam may irradiate the pelvis (i.e. those between the diaphragm and knees), or nuclear medicine scans, the referring clinician should enter the relevant pregnancy details on the request card on any female of reproductive age, or state 'not known'. Further checks must be made by the 'operator' at the time of examination (the pregnancy status may also have changed in the interval). Responses are listed as one of the following:

1   No possibility of pregnancy.
2   Patient definitely or probably pregnant.
3   Pregnancy cannot be excluded: low-risk procedure.
4   Pregnancy cannot be excluded: high-risk procedure.

The risk of the procedure is classified as low, intermediate or high-risk:

Low dose procedure (< 1 mGy)	Intermediate dose procedure (1- 10 mGy)	High risk procedure (> 10 mGy)
Extremity X-rays	Barium enema	CT abdomen
CXR	IVU	CT pelvis
AXR	Nuclear medicine bone scan	CT chest/abdomen/pelvis
V/Q scan	Lumbar spine X-ray	Nuclear medicine myocardial scan
Mammography	PET scan	SPECT scan
Thoracic spine X-ray		PET-CT
MAG-3 renal scan		
Nuclear medicine thyroid scan		
CTPA		
CT chest		

If the response is '1' all examinations can be performed. If '2' the radiologist and clinician need to discuss the relevant risks and benefits also giving consideration to delaying the examination or using techniques such as US or MRI. If the answer is '3', and the patient's next menstrual period is not overdue, all low dose and intermediate dose procedures can be performed. For the majority of diagnostic procedures (up to 1 mGy) the risks of inducing a childhood cancer are low (< 1/10 000) and much less than the natural risk (1 in 500). Thus all such examinations can be performed as long as they are justified and ALARP principles are followed. The low risk of childhood cancer is not sufficient to justify pregnancy termination. If the answer is '4', procedures > 10 mGy should not be performed as, even in the first few weeks of pregnancy, the risk of inducing a childhood cancer is deemed too high and such examinations should be avoided if possible. There is a negligible risk of causing radiation-induced hereditary disease in the descendants of the unborn child.

Cases of inadvertent radiation exposure may result if the patient denies being pregnant (deliberately or unknowingly), or was not asked the relevant question. In all such cases an investigation must be performed by the medical physics expert in accordance with local IR(ME)R procedures. It may also be relevant to formal report this as an incident of 'much greater than intended exposure'.

Further reading:
* www.rcr.ac.uk/docs/radiology/pdf/HPA_Diagnostic_Pregnancy.pdf.

15

The increased availability of CT and the improved quality of imaging, combined with government led targets and guidelines, mean that there are increasing demands on the radiology department both within hours and out-of-hours. Examples of national frameworks include NICE guidelines on CT imaging post-head injury and the National Stroke Strategy for the early diagnosis of stroke. The RCR recently acknowledged the need for out-of-hours radiology cover with the statement '… clinical radiology is now so central to the management of so many patients that its delivery can no longer be confined to *office hours*'.

Diagnostically, outsourcing via teleradiology is a potential method of providing out-of-hours radiology cover 24 hours a day, 7 days a week, however, it brings certain disadvantages along with it (*see* viva question 12). Nevertheless, teleradiology is at best only a partial solution, as there are certain radiological procedures that require the radiologist to be physically present within the department: all ultrasounds, all interventional procedures (including angiograms / angioplasty, nephrostomies), and any image-guided procedure (such as insertion of a chest drain or intra-abdominal drain). The role of diagnostic angiography may be partially taken over by improvements in CT-angiography and (to a lesser extent out of hours) MR-angiography.

Ultimately, patient safety and optimal patient management must be placed first, and recognition of the important role that diagnostic and interventional radiology plays in the provision of modern medical care means that 24-hour cover by a radiologist is essential. In providing such cover, consideration needs to be given to the European working-time directive, which states that doctors in training should be working a maximum 48-hour week (from August 2009); consultants can voluntarily opt out of these limits, but new jobs cannot be advertised which incorporate more than these hours. Furthermore, formal radiology rotas need to be supported by appropriate nursing and radiography staff. The RCR recommends that there should be a clear policy on out-of-hours radiology for each department on which examinations (and in which clinical situations) influence immediate medical management. Referral protocols should be in place for non-core procedures +/- investigations, thus seriously ill patients are imaged immediately and non-urgent cases do not overwhelm the system – in particular, imaging should not be performed out of hours when it would be better dealt with during normal working hours when all appropriate staff are available. It should also be made clear what is and what is not possible to be provided in and out of hours at the local hospital, and procedures need to be in place for reporting risk management and other issues of clinical governance.

Further reading

- RCR. *Standards for providing a 24-hour interventional radiology service*. London: RCR; 2008.
- RCR. *Standards for providing a 24-hour diagnostic radiology service*. London: RCR; 2009.

Bibliography

- Chapman S, Nakielny R, editors. *Aids to Radiological Differential Diagnosis*. 4th ed. Philadelphia, PA: Saunders; 2003.
- Dahnert W, editor. *Radiology Review Manual*. 6th ed. Philadelphia, PA: Lippincott Williams & Wilkins; 2007.
- De Lacey G, Morley S, Berman LH, editors. *The Chest X-Ray: a survival guide*. London: Elsevier, Saunders; 2007.
- Gore RM, Levine MS, editors. *Textbook of Gastrointestinal Radiology*. 3rd ed. Philadelphia, PA: Saunders; 2007.
- Kessel D, Robertson I, editors. *Interventional Radiology: a survival guide*. 2nd ed. London: Elsevier, Churchill-Livingstone; 2005.
- Kuhn JP, Slovis TL, Haller JO, editors. *Caffey's Pediatric Diagnostic Imaging*. 10th ed. St Louis, MO: Mosby; 2003.
- Moore KL, Dalley AF, editors. *Clinically Oriented Anatomy*. 5th ed. Philadelphia, PA: Lippincott Williams and Wilkins; 2005.
- Raby N, Berman LH, De Lacey G, editors. *Accident & Emergency Radiology*. 2nd ed. London: Elsevier, Saunders; 2005.
- Royal College of Radiologists. *Making the Best Use of Clinical Radiology Services: Referral Guidelines*. 6th ed. London: Royal College of Radiologists; 2007.
- Rubin M, Safdieh JE, editors. *Netter's Concise Neuroanatomy*. Philadelphia, PA: Saunders; 2007.

Index of answers

6   Prematurity versus post-maturity
7   Extra-dural haematoma
8   Crohn's disease versus UC
9   CF associations
10 CT investigation
11 Radiologists' roles
12 Gallstones
13 Fluoroscopic swallow investigation
14 'White out' at CXR
15 Obstetric US
16 CXR artefacts
17 Fracture descriptions
18 Radiology investigations and breast feeding
19 Meckel's diverticulum
20 Polyhydramnios
21 Breast US
22 Bone scintigraphy
23 Croup
24 Free air under the diaphragm
25 Investigation of anaemia
26 Investigation of PV bleeding
27 Investigation of prostate cancer
28 Rheumatoid arthritis versus osteoarthritis
29 Renal calculi
30 Hilar lymphadenopathy
31 Neonatal CXR
32 Investigation of trauma
33 NAI
34 Positron emission tomography
35 Ultrasound
36 Mammography
37 Paget's disease
38 Hyperparathyroidism
39 Post-pneumonectomy CXR
40 Elbow ossification centres
41 V/Q scan
42 Achilles tendon rupture
43 Investigation of adrenal adenoma
44 Pneumothorax
45 Investigation of claudication
46 Cavernous sinus anatomy
47 Intracranial calcification
48 'White out' at CXR
49 Bone metastases
50 Radioactive tracer injections

CHAPTER 6 EMIs

1   Upper limb trauma
2   Investigation of anaemia
3   Radiological signs
4   What examination is being performed? Part 1
5   Radiological findings in the phakomatoses
6   Inflammatory bowel disease
7   What examination is being performed? Part 2
8   Investigation of abdominal pain
9   Chest pathology
10 Normal anatomical variants at CXR
11 Haematuria
12 Phaeochromocytomas
13 CT Head examination
14 Arthritides
15 Lower limb trauma
16 Chest X-ray
17 Breast imaging
18 Neonatal radiology
19 Bone tumours
20 Abdominal X-ray

CHAPTER 7 SBAs

1   Investigation of PE
2   Pulmonary hamartoma
3   Radiation dose
4   Investigation of AAA
5   Investigation of anaemia
6   Abdominal perforation
7   Investigation of RUQ pain
8   Inguinal hernia
9   Investigation of UTI in a child
10 Investigation of biliary tract stones
11 Fluoroscopic swallow
12 Radiation dose
13 TIA management
14 Investigation of post-menopausal bleed
15 Fractured neck of femur
16 Osteoarthritis
17 CT Hounsfield units
18 Kartagener's syndrome
19 Sarcoid
20 CT in stroke
21 Tylosis
22 Slipped upper femoral epiphysis

23 Situs relationships
24 Respiratory distress syndrome
25 Investigation of a renal mass
26 Nuclear medicine renal imaging
27 Erect CXR
28 Sigmoid volvulus
29 Investigation of microscopic haematuria
30 Testicular torsion
31 Popular radiological investigations
32 Renal angiomyolipoma
33 Normal pressure hydrocephalus
34 Pseudohypoparathyroidism
35 Hypertrophic osteoarthropathy
36 Paget's disease
37 Pectus excavatum
38 Ankylosing spondylitis
39 Cardiac anatomy at CXR
40 CT colonography
41 Investigation of back pain
42 Rotator cuff injury
43 Elbow trauma
44 Rickets
45 Radiation dose
46 Slipped upper femoral epiphysis
47 Investigation of trauma
48 Intussusception
49 Ewing's sarcoma
50 Bone metastases

CHAPTER 8 SAQs

1 Radiology request form information
2 Fracture mimics
3 Pericardial calcification
4 Cervical spine trauma
5 Head injury
6 CXR in rheumatoid arthritis
7 Cavitating chest lesions
8 Congenital CNS infection
9 Hydrocephalus
10 Bronchiectasis
11 Contraindications to MRI
12 Honeycombing of the lung
13 Osteopenia
14 Splenomegaly
15 Thyroid enlargement
16 Eosinophilic pneumonia

17 Fluorosis
18 Raised left hemidiaphragm
19 Pulmonary oedema
20 Extrinsic allergic alveolitis
21 Bone scintigraphy
22 Avascular necrosis of the hip
23 'Cannonball' lung metastases
24 Small bowel obstruction
25 Sacro-ilitis
26 Pulmonary arterial enlargement
27 Upper zone lung fibrosis
28 Signs of abdominal perforation
29 Unilateral lung translucency
30 Ring-enhancing brain lesion

CHAPTER 9 VIVA VOCE

1 Contrast agents
2 Paediatric radiation protection
3 Breast screening
4 Radiology and the trauma patient
5 Radiation protection
6 Radiology and non-accidental injury
7 Advantages and disadvantages of PACS systems
8 Functional imaging
9 CT / MRI of head injury
10 Radiation dose
11 Skills mix
12 Advantages and disadvantages of teleradiology
13 Reporting of unexpected findings
14 Radiation in pregnancy
15 24-hour radiology cover in the hospital

Index